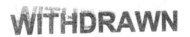

"So he got even with me at last, in the only way he could, for all my sarcastic attacks: he didn't even mention the recipe I sent him for *sauerkraus*."

—Karl Kraus

"Nigh to being the only civilized thing, that is to say, the only readable book, afforded the English reader by this curious figure from an epoch still known to us as Hapsburg."

—Henry James

"A lovely book, a work of genius. I am sending him some peaches."

—Nellie Melba

Freud's Own Cookbook

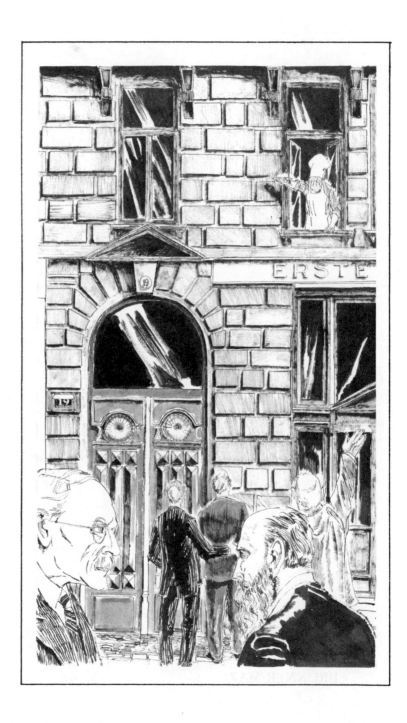

FREUD'S OWN COOKBOOK

Edited by
James Hillman
and Charles Boer

Illustrated by Jeff Fisher

BRUNNER/MAZEL *Publishers* • *New York*

Library of Congress Cataloging in Publication Data

Hillman, James, 1926–.
  Freud's own cookbook.

  Includes index.
  1. Cookery. 2. Freud, Sigmund, 1856–1939. 3. Psychoanalysts. I.
Boer, Charles, 1939–.
II. Title.
TX652.H545   1984   641.5   84-47579
ISBN 0-87630-497-8

Designer: C. Linda Dingler

First Brunner/Mazel, Inc. Edition, 1987.

BRUNNER/MAZEL, INC.
19 Union Square
New York, New York 10003

Manufactured in the United States of America

10 9 8 7 6 5 4 3 2 1

TABLE CONTENTS

ACKNOWLEDGMENTS

The editors wish to express their gratitude to the Sigmund Freud Archives for not considering the manuscript of this book important enough to be put under lock and key and thus not impeding in any way its being made available to readers in this century.

We would also like to thank Patricia Berry, A. K. Donohue, Wolfgang Giegerich, Grazia Giorgi, William Kotzwinkle, Jay Livernois, Maidena McLerran, and Robert Rosenthal for their assistance.

EDITORS' NOTE

Throughout the text, we have kept Freud's own spelling of German words for such dishes as *Sulz, Bauernschinken, Stollen,* etc., although he often uses Viennese, Moravian, Yiddish, and even Hungarian dialect spellings instead of the standard High German. The recipes written in England, late in his life, seem especially prone to such variations. A study of these discrepancies in spelling, and the serious misconceptions they have wrought in the dissemination of Freud's thought in English, is being prepared separately.

Freud's Own Cookbook

INTRODUCTION

Joy! pleasure! delight! What a clarion call those complex words are for humanity still. It is public knowledge that before the turn of the century, while I was barely in my forties, I had already given up sexual joy. Yet fate so willed that my death was postponed for at least another forty years. Where then was pleasure to be gained? What did the libido want—moreover, what did this sexual abstinence say about the libido itself? Could I have been wrong in regard to its origin in sexuality (could I have been wrong about sexuality itself?)? Yes, the principle of life is Eros—but might not the primary organization of the erotic be oral and remain oral through the final meal?

My later years have convinced me that this indeed is the case. Theory-construction by my disciples must give more attention to oral eroticism. This is not being done. My theories, based on discoveries in the eighties and nineties of the last century, have become unconscious recipes. We cannot ignore that our early cases were plump well-fed ladies and gentlemen who had themselves three to four hearty meals a day. In Vienna we all ate well. There was sexual repression, of course, but certainly not oral (the *Sulz* and the *Knödels,* the *geröstetes Leber* and *kalte Aufschnitt, Salzstangls, Milchrahmstrudel,* the *Stollen* and *Schnecken* from the bakeries, the *Schnitzels mit Erdapfelstock,* and the green wine from the hills!).

Alas, all this was neglected by the next generation . . .
so many Americans, so many medical men who had rarely
eaten outside their miserable hospital cafeterias. I tried to
warn against the influence of the medical in my essay *The
Question of Lay Analysis* (1926). I knew that if psychoanalysis fell into the hands of the medical profession, the
culinary art would soon disappear from psychoanalysis and
with it all its cultural roots. Doctors do not eat well, and
they have sublimated their oral frustrations into dire warn-
ings: against rich foods now called "fatty," against the zest
of salt and the delight of sugars, against red meats and
sweet cream, against sauces, the very acme of the culinary
art. Against even pastries! Instead we are to eat like cows
and horses—raw vegetables, brown grains, balanced
meals. Balanced diets produce unbalanced minds! Meals
accompanied by pills instead of compotes, pickles, condi-
ments, and wines! It is no wonder dietary supplements become necessary when diet itself becomes as deprived, as
depraved, as that which my medical colleagues now foist
upon an orally repressed, and so, discontented civilization.

Malnutrition: that is the problem. Traumatic neuroses
are being perpetrated upon the victims of civilization every
day in the lunchroom, the restaurant, and the home.
Snacks, dips, Cokes, and burgers: this is the true psychopathology of everyday life—not slips and inadvertencies of
the pen and the tongue, not little misreadings and forget-
tings, but bad food. Of course anxiety prevails. What I said
in 1926 in *Inhibitions, Symptoms, and Anxiety* has been
solidly confirmed by history: anxiety is the reaction to dan-
ger and produces repression. Food has become dangerous.
We defend against it in every possible way—especially with
diets which are simply inhibitions—and subsequently we
suffer symptoms of every sort which psychoanalysis still
insists upon tracing to sexual origins.

The evidence is all around us that psychoanalysis is on
the wrong track, or let us say, has persisted too long in the

paths, once new, that I laid down so many years ago. A host of new hysterical disorders, symptoms, and anxieties greets us at every turn: bulemia, obesity, food allergies, anorexia nervosa, diet fads, vitamin and mineral addictions (imagine desiring kelp and dolomite!), food phobias, carcinogenic paranoias, to say nothing of the nostalgias for health food—the wild rice, berries, and bone meal of the primal horde, our archaic ancestors.

But why, I must ask myself, does the oral origin of the neuroses only now force itself upon my attention? How can I account for such a prolonged misreading?

We do not need to wander far afield to discover an answer. The great questions that have persistently plagued psychoanalysis, and which it was always courageous enough to encounter, thereby setting it off on new paths and correcting its old ones, are to be found within psychoanalysis itself. And the one answer to all misreadings, to all inadequately conceived theories of reality, we have from the start: the pleasure principle.

The instinctual Id, that ever-vital source of pleasure, "is the psyche proper" (as I said in 1926). Psychological life must be pleasurable, and psychology, too, an instinctual joy, else my name is not Freud.

Owing, however, to the vicissitudes of the instincts, that one instinct can replace or reinforce another, the sexual instinct with its modes of pleasurable gratification at times usurps more than its share, succeeding in disguising the very roots of pleasure itself. For its base is oral; it loves to eat. The child comes before the man, the tongue before the penis, the mouth before the vulva, phylogenetically and ontogenetically. And today the statistical rise in the incidence of oral sexuality gives the lie to the theory that the oral is a "partial" drive, a foreplay. No, these sexual acts with the mouth are attempts on the part of the oral drive to incorporate the genital into its libidinal source from which the genital emerged in late childhood, forcing the

mouth into a prolonged latency period, sometimes resulting in the food disorders of early adolescence: obesity and
anorexia (see below, "Psychoculinary Development and the
Eating Crisis at Puberty"). One need only look at the food
terms and simulated food fragrances that have recently
been given to genital douches, suppositories, and sexual
stimulators to see how overtly sexual gratifications derive
from oral pleasures. In the beginning comes the mouth.
Anatomy is destiny. What do women want? They want
lunch! a good dinner! an honest wine list!

A clue to the primacy of food—a clue before which all
theoretical obduracy must bow—was granted me by my
own daughter, Anna, in the autumn of 1897, at the age of
one and a half. "During the night she called out a whole
menu in her sleep: 'Stwawbewwies, wild stwawbewwies,
omblet, pudden.' "

This dream, famous now because of my having reported it to Fliess and in two of my books on dreams, states
beyond questioning how culturally elevated and lasci-
viously delicious is the unconscious mind of even the tiniest child. Hardly past infancy, Anna, who was destined
too to lay her head upon my couch for a prolonged analysis
and then to become one of the great mentors of the psychoanalytic movement, had as her first recorded dream
this superb menu of fulfilled oral pleasure.

Had I looked less intellectually and more with a true
clinical eye at my own dreams years ago, I might have seen
that the mouth was staring me in the face quite literally.
The very first dream of my self-analysis with its brilliant
interpretation that set the course of psychoanalysis ever
after has me examining a certain "Irma's" oral cavity. In
that dream I look straight down her throat. Such a *Wich-
tigtuer* I was then, having to impress with the finesse of my
interpretation that I forgot the first rule of a good doctor:
alleviate the symptoms. And Irma in the dream sure had
them. She says: "If only you knew what pains I've got now

in my throat and stomach and abdomen—it's choking me." Clearly she needed—and I, the dreamer needed— some help with an eating problem. But my theory of the li- bido utterly ignored Irma's inflamed digestive tract.

Or take a later dream of mine where I go into the kitchen in search of some pudding. Three women are there standing around. One is making *Knödels* (dumplings). She tells me I must wait till she is ready. Already then I under- stood these women as the Three Fates and said so in my great dream book. But I considered "making dumplings a queer occupation for a Fate, and one that cried out for an explanation." Here, in these pages, is the explanation; Fate has finally yielded up the pudding, this cookbook; psycho- analysis comes home to the kitchen.

Yet a further clue was shown me during this same pe- riod, this one by my own body. For during the intense scrutiny of my self-analysis which I reported on regularly by letter to Fliess in Berlin, I observed: "Under the influ- ence of the analysis my heart-trouble is now often replaced by stomach-trouble."

My stomach was drawing my attention but I did not lis- ten, so bent was I upon the sexual theory. Was my thirst for fame through scandal—the sexual theory being the surest path—the factor that blinded me to my Anna's dream, to Irma's choking, and my own stomach? Was it the influence on me of ancient Jewish tradition that thought too much of food and too little of sex? (Though my father was out of a Chassidic milieu and recorded my first name in the fam- ily Bible as Schlomo, I had no Jewish education except eat- ing religiously.) Or was it the theory of repression itself which required that the content of the repressed could not be what was then on everybody's daily mind in bourgeois Vienna: the buying, preparing, and eating of food?

And could the affliction suffered in my own person and so pointedly located in the oral cavity, bringing me inex- orably toward my end in London (whose food, fortunately, is hardly palatable), be yet one more indication of this complex state of affairs?

However we now reconstruct the case of psychoanalytic theory and of its founder, yours truly, Professor Sigmund Freud, one certainty does stand forth: analysis will remain interminable and stoicism prevail in Freudianism unless the pleasures of the oral cavity with its surrounding membranes and olfactory apparatus be given their instinctual due.

So, in extreme old age, I have assembled this book; and like my other works it serves both manifest and latent purposes. First, it shows I did not, as biographers have untruly reported, keep Martha in the kitchen while I retired to the *Schreibstube* to write those interminable papers which have given food for thought to a century of "Freudians." No, not food for thought, thought for food—I, too, was in the kitchen, sometimes alone, sometimes side by side with her sister Minna Bernays, my noble sister-in-law. *Ménage à trois.* Early on, I was a liberated man, giving outlet to what old Fliess and Weininger (and later Jung and Adler in their plagiaristic way) came to call bisexuality or inner femininity.

The public has been misguided about those evenings in the *Schreibstube.* Yes, I was writing, but writing what? Cases and theories, of course. But also rewriting the dishes I garnered from teachers and colleagues and from notes I had taken down during the day as I sat hour after hour unobserved behind the talking heads of patients who freely associated some of the most unusual recipes that one with an interest such as mine will ever be granted the fortune to hear.

There is, therefore, an unevenness in what follows. Different times, different sauces; and my fluctuating moods are evident in these pages. But a cookbook should not be composed with that attention to style necessary for a scientific theory to win its way in the world. Moreover, this book serves to free me from the burdened prose of my other books, that style in which I have been forced to write ever since I was praised, at age seventeen, when my German professor compared me to Herder and for which I was commended by Thomas Mann, no less. Here I have not had to construct a work in emulation of the great literary masters whom I so admired. Here I could reconstruct, or just not "struct" at all, and write as I liked.

Here, too, I can make corrections that have been needed for years and years; for instance, the irritating interpretation of a casual remark, since become notorious, that I let pass one evening after a very good *Sauerbraten mit Eiernudeln:* "Sometimes a cigar is only a cigar." I was simply referring to the oral delight of smoking which was then being subtly undermined by my followers—far too many of whom were nonsmokers—by giving to the cigar a genital significance. This interpretation of cigar betrays an unfortunate, because unrecognized, cigar-envy and a desire to castrate the father who smokes for pleasure.

The irony will not escape the reader that precisely by means of a cookbook I am able to take revenge upon my adulators by revising those theories—wrested with such struggle from the bedrock of my psyche—which in their hands have become simplified into formula and denigrated as Freudian "cookbook" psychology. Only genuine recipes can cure psychoanalysis of its cookbookism.♦

♦ In the margin of this page of the manuscript appear several notes by Freud suggesting to himself a possible title for this book. We give the German original for these, as well as our translation, in the order in which he wrote them at the side of the page: 1) *Die Freud des Essens* ("The Joy of Eating"); 2) *Die Freud des Kochens* ("The Joy of Cooking"); 3) *Der Freud des Kochens* ("The Freud of Cooking"). After the last one, but in a hand that may have been Martha's, is written, *"Ja!"*—*The Editors.*

Further than these theoretical corrections, this book serves as a complement to my *Autobiographical Study* (1925). That was written, as every reader knows, partly in self-justification, and therefore had to omit much of my interests, my nature, and my daily life. The present collection also offers the opportunity to bring back old friends, their faces as we ate together and the foods we shared. All those strange fates, strange deaths: Tausk, Ferenczi, Reich, Abraham. How mad we all were. So, this book is an essay in reminiscence, like Jung's late work; it is my *Memories, Creams, Confections:* a recollection of the old days in the Vienna circle and beyond. Enough has been recorded in the famous minutes of what we said; yet not one word of what we ate.

It is as well, finally, a contribution to the pleasure principle of everyday life. It seems almost a century ago that the psychopathology of everyday life was explored and analyzed. Enough about that. At my age who wants to hear of trouble? Problems, I have had enough. But a good dish—tomorrow's menu—the possibility of yet one more wish fulfilled—such is the source and satisfaction of a long life well lived.

NOTES

"while I was barely in my forties . . ."; letter to Fliess, 31 October 1897, *The Origins of Psycho-Analysis, Letters to Wilhelm Fliess, Drafts and Notes: 1887–1902, by Sigmund Freud,* Ed. Marie Bonaparte, Anna Freud, Ernst Kris (New York, Basic Books, 1954), p. 227.

"is the psyche proper"; *The Question of Lay Analysis,* trans. Nancy Procter-Gregg (London: Imago, 1947), p. 15.

"During the night she cried out"; letter to Fliess, 31 October 1897, *Letters to Wilhelm Fliess,* op. cit.

"If only you knew what pains"; *The Interpretation of Dreams,*

trans. J. Strachey (London: Allen & Unwin, 1954), p. 107.
"Or take a later dream of mine"; ibid., pp. 204–205.
"Under the influence of the analysis"; letter to Fliess, 31 October 1897.

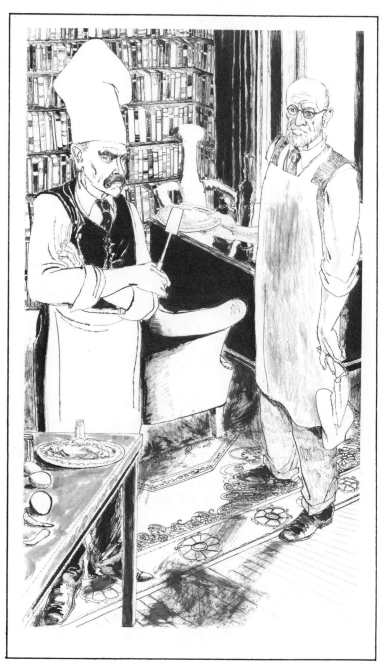

Scrambled Jaureggs

I.

EARLIEST MEMORIES

Especially Momovers
and Mesmer-Icing

*"You're a lucky mother! Someday the whole world
will talk about this little fellow."*

Spoken by a stranger in a pastry shop
to the mother of four-year-old Sigmund.
Quoted by Anna Freud Bernays,
in *Freud as We Knew Him,* ed.
Hendrik M. Ruitenbeek

MOMOVERS

I remember Momovers, but have not had any, alas, since 1930, when my mother, Amalia (born Nathansohn), died at the age of ninety-five. Without her, I know, I shall manage only a few more years. What a woman, always joyful (*Freudvoll*), always sharp-witted. When she called me, even in front of strangers, *"mein goldener Sigi,"* was it out of genuine affection or to get my goat? Although an ocean of differences lay between us, I am sure I received many little traits from her, like my vanity about dressing and about photographs. A few weeks before she died, when her photograph appeared in the newspapers, her comment was, "A bad reproduction; it makes me look a hundred!" None of that matters anymore. I remember her Momovers, light and fresh and golden as the dawn.

> Mix 1 cup of flour with a handful of oat flakes. Add 1 tsp. salt, 1 cup milk, 1 egg yolk. Add 1 stiffly beaten egg white. Put in greased Momover pans (use Popover pans if not available), and bake in 425° oven for half an hour, or until the puffs "mom" over.

NOTES
"Mein goldener Sigi"; Ernest Jones, *The Life and Work of Sigmund Freud* (New York: Basic Books, 1953), vol. 1, p. 3.
"A bad reproduction . . ."; ibid.

CHRISTMAS DINNER WITH THE FREUDS

Amalia ignored the Jewish feasts but celebrated Christmas and Easter. For many years, even after I had my own children, we would all go to Mother's flat on Christmas for a dinner of roast goose, candied fruits, cakes, and punch.

First, she would scrub the goose thoroughly with a brush in order to render the oil more easily. Then, after rinsing and wiping the inside dry, she would cram it with her priceless stuffing: potatoes mashed and seasoned with a chopped truffle that had been cooked in a little white wine. To this was added 1 tsp. of crisp diced bacon. (Amalia observed no dietary taboos—far from it! She came from that wild, almost barbarous land, East Galicia.) The goose was cooked in a medium oven until brown and tender. It was always served with applesauce.

NOTE

"Amalia ignored the Jewish feasts"; Martin Freud, *Sigmund Freud, Man and Father* (New York: Vanguard, 1958), p. 11.

FILLETTE MIGNON

When I was a little boy, just after we moved to Vienna from Moravia, my father was mysteriously visited by a shriveled-up Italian woman in the first stages of senile dementia. She gave him this recipe, and it is the oldest in my collection. What else she revealed to him he never said, except that she had been in her youth the nymphlike Italian girl, Mignon, described by Goethe (in *Wilhelm Meister's Lehrjahre*), a girl of ambiguous sexuality and subject to hysterical seizures. The impressions that such mysterious visits make upon an observant little boy! I remained fascinated all my life with Fillette Mignon, ordering it wherever I could. When I was awarded the famous Goethe Prize for my writing ability, I told the audience in Frankfurt how much I, like Goethe, loved Fillette Mignon, but that Goethe never revealed his love, he being such a "careful concealer." What he concealed was what this woman told my father, who in turned concealed it from me. It was this recipe, tender, nymphlike, Italian, and a touch hysterical.

> You will need fillet steaks of at least 1 inch thickness. Heat 2 tbs. olive oil in a pan. Brown a clove of crushed garlic in the oil, then discard the garlic. Add 1 or 2 tomatoes, thinly sliced, to the pan. Season with chopped fresh oregano, and salt and pepper. Add 2 tbs. white wine and cook tomatoes for about 5 minutes. Meanwhile, put 2 tbs. oil and 2 tbs. butter in a skillet. When hot, sear the fillets for a few minutes on each side. Quickly add 2 tbs. cognac to the pan and continue cooking for 2 minutes. Season with salt and pepper. Serve the Fillettes Mignons with the tomato slices on top.

NOTE

Cf. *The Freud/Jung Letters,* ed. William McGuire, trans. Ralph Manheim and R. F. C. Hull (Princeton: Princeton University Press, 1974), p. 388.

THE GISELA COMPLEX, OR COOKING WITH WINE

My writings say next to nothing about alcoholism, and my life was unusually sober in that regard (of course, not virulently sober like Jung—Ferenczi and I only got Jung to break the pledge on the eve of our departure together for America). And Bleuler! Why, the entire staff at Burghölzli took the pledge; what the patients did remains unreported.

I drank the local wines wherever we traveled, but as I wrote my friend Fliess, "any drop of alcohol makes me stupid," and both fainting fits that happened when I was with Jung came over me after I had drunk some wine. My illness in 1912 was due in part to drinking wine in the Tyrol, and I felt better, in Rome that fall, "after almost renouncing the Roman red wine," as I wrote Binswanger.

Wine brought back the memory of that stupendous drunk, at age sixteen, when I vomited violently and fell down unconscious to be nursed through the night by the mother of the girl for whom I had conceived a secret passion, Gisela Flüss. This has been the greatest secret that every one of my followers has tried to decipher. My girl, my Gisela—how I suppressed all associations to her, her name, the color yellow of the dress she wore. Probably the dyspnea I often later suffered at meals is a hysterical reminiscence of the mention by her mother at mealtimes of this wild Thracian beauty with long black hair.

Yet deeper in the Gisela complex lies the imago of her mother, Frau Flüss. The phonetic echo of her name, so close to Fliess, my dearest friend for years, and that both their names are variations upon the word "flow," again points to the god of wine, Dionysus, who no more enters my work than drunkenness entered my consciousness—except for Gisela and her mother.

I had actually "translated" my esteem for Frau Flüss to the daughter—and said so in a moment of indiscretion in a letter I afterward tried to recover and suppress. No, it was not my mother complex that truly attracted me—one look at Amalia would clarify that misapprehension; it was Gisela's mother. The suppressing of this youthful passion all these years has given a false twist to the complex of mother-love. Oedipus is not the complex, Gisela is. A man loves his mother-in-law. It is the mother-daughter imago in the woman, the mother translated into a daughter, that holds the ultimate power over a man's erotic destiny. So I could never get drunk again, never let the Dionysian flow directly into my work, or pay attention to alcoholic patients, for fear of suffering the reminiscence of the Flüsses, mother and daughter. Instead of alcohol, I preferred wine sublimated in cooking jugged hare, bordelaise sauces, consommé with sherry. . . .

NOTES

"any drop of alcohol makes me stupid"; letter to Fliess, 19 April 1896, quoted in Max Schur, *Freud: Living and Dying* (New York: Inter University Press, 1972), p. 98.

"after almost renouncing the Roman red wine"; cited, Max Schur, op. cit., p. 265.

"My girl, my Gisela"; see Ronald W. Clark, *Freud: The Man and the Cause* (New York: Random House, 1980), ch. 2.

FECHNER'S BAUERNSCHINKEN
(Country Ham)

"Our entire civilization is nothing more than a product of the activity of the stomach."

"The whole body is really but an excrement of the stomach which is set around by the body like a crust, a fur to keep it soft and warm."

"The stomach is the alpha and omega of creation."
"The happiest being would be an infinite stomach that never filled and could eat forever."

—Gustav Theodor Fechner (alias Dr. Mises), *Stapelia Mixta* (1824)

My reading in "old Fechner," as I often endearingly referred to him, taught me many things. I willingly admit that basic psychoanalytic ideas can already be found in his work: that the mind has its own energy, that the unconscious is a distinct region, that life is dominated by the pleasure/unpleasure principle. But I wish now, in the light of this, my final book, that I had paid even closer attention to him.

Fechner was a curious man, both a famous exact scientist and a mystical metaphysician—is that why, though I never knew him, I felt so close to him?

He appreciated the significance of dreams even before my discoveries saw the light of day. During a morbid depression once, lasting three years, Fechner suffered from photophobia and would not go out of doors without blue glasses. He suffered as well from alimentary disorders so that he allowed himself only the blandest of diets: then it was that a woman friend dreamed of preparing him a *Bauernschinken,* a ham cured in lemon juice and Rhine wine. She made the dish, carried it to his place, whereupon he, against his better judgment, ate it. His appetite was restored and Fechner went on to live another forty-four years.

The hero of this cure, however, is neither the woman, the dream, nor Gustav Theodor Fechner. The hero, as always, is a ham.

If you cannot buy your *Bauernschinken* already cured this way, put cloves in a ham (3 to 7 lbs.) and marinate for several hours in a cup or two of German white wine and the juice of a lemon. Turn the ham often. Before cooking, spread German mustard over the top and then lay thin slices of lemon over this, until the ham is completely covered (the lemon helps fight photophobia). The ham should be cooked in a shallow pan, with the marinade and an additional cup of wine for about two hours in a 325° oven. Serve with the lemon slices and pour the pan juices on top.

NOTE

Stapelia Mixta, reprinted in *Die Freud des Essens,* ed. Herbert Heckmann (Munich: Hanser Verlag, 1979), pp. 410–414.

MESMER-ICING

The strange treatments I used in the early days—hypno-
tism, suggestion, my attempts with cocaine, probing intimate sexual reminiscences with a patient, often a woman,
prone on a couch—drew odious comparisons with an earlier Viennese physician, Franz Anton Mesmer (1734–
1815). He discovered "animal magnetism" and treated
people by throwing them into trances and waving a thin
iron rod that supposedly rearranged for the benefit of the
patient the cosmic energies of the universe, "a subtle invisible effluvia," as he called it. But that was only icing on
the cake. There was more.

The invisible effluvia, however, which, Mesmer said,
causes illness and also cures it, has nothing whatsoever to
do with the unconscious. Nor do the laws that supposedly
govern magnetism have anything to do with the laws determining the psyche. Moreover, my theory of the libido as
the energy of Eros is to be distinguished absolutely from
Mesmer's magnetic fluidum and its erotic effects. *Kein
Vergleich!*

How patients love charlatans! Mesmer employed hand-
some young men as his assistants, and he dressed in a lilac
coat of silk, walked up and down among a crowd of en-
tranced, enchanted patients, mostly female, all placed
around a circular oaken tub (the *baquet*) in which empty
bottles were geometrically arranged for collecting and dis-
tributing the magnetic fluidum. Sometimes he made
passes with his hands over their bodies, seated opposite
them foot to foot, knee to knee, even touching their lower
abdomens. (The analytical couch put a stop to such heed-
less intimacy.)

Compared with the scientific rigor of psychoanalytic
methods and the efforts we employ to test its recipes, Mes-

mer's sugary charlatanism should be likened not to me and my authentic discoveries but to Wilhelm Reich, another purveyor of cosmic egg white.

I give the recipe for Mesmer-Icing, therefore, only so that the reader may compare it with my own Wish-Fulfillment Icing, and so that he may observe how, with so much messy theorizing going on, I have to strenuously defend the borders of our discipline, psychoanalysis, from charlatanism of every kind.

> In a saucepan combine all the sugar you want (1 cup will do a cake), about the same amount of water, 1 tbs. corn syrup, and a dash of salt. Boil, stirring gently, until it thickens. Cool. In top of your Double-Bleuler, melt all the chocolate you want (5 oz. will do a cake) with 1 tsp. strong coffee per oz. of chocolate. Stir in about the same amount of butter as chocolate. Pour out a glass of rum and add half to the chocolate. Sip the other half while stirring chocolate mixture into cooled syrup. When cool, blend in 1/3 cup whipped cream. Stir until both icing and you feel smooth. After Mesmer-Icing the cake, sprinkle the top with silver jimmies.

MALE EEL BOILED IN BEER

My first sight of a southern civilization came in March 1876, when, as a student at the University of Vienna, I was sent by Professor Carl Claus on a research excursion to his Zoological Experimental Station at Trieste to study a problem that had puzzled science since the days of Aristotle, namely, the gonadic structure of eels. As I wrote in my paper for Claus, "No one has ever found a mature male eel— no one has yet seen the testes of the eel, in spite of innumerable efforts through the centuries." I dissected four hundred eels, and found a small lobed organ in many of them, which, I surmised, was the missing testes. On microscopic examination, I found the histological structure of the organ such that it had to be an immature form of testes. To think that for so many years people could not find something as plain and simple as that. I soon realized that I would have to apply my gonadal research to even bigger fish.

To make male eel steamed in beer, you must first be sure you have a male eel. Cut it into little pieces and boil them in a pot with a glass of beer and some chopped shallots. Season the liquid with salt and pepper and then thicken it with a little arrowroot. If there are ladies present, cover the eel with parsley.

NOTES

"my paper for Claus"; "Beobachtungen über Gestaltung und feineren Bau der als Hoden beschriebenen Lappenorgane des Aals," *S. B. Akad. Wiss.* (Vienna: *Math.-Naturwiss. Kl.*, 1877) Abt., Bd. 75, p. 15.
"No one has ever found . . ."; cited, Jones, *Life and Work,* vol. 1, p. 42.

SCRAMBLED JAUREGGS

Julius Wagner-Jauregg, for such was the doctor's name, was my school friend and rival. Ever scrambling for position and notoriety, Julius came to hold the most prestigious psychiatric position in the entire Austro-Hungarian Empire, when I was not even a regular faculty member. He was awarded the first and only Nobel Prize given to a psychiatrist; I had to rest content with the Goethe Prize (and who outside Frankfurt ever heard of it?). Julius' head decorates the 500-Schilling note; my name was not even to be commemorated on the house where I lived until 1954! My innovations with cocaine achieved nothing; Julius was immensely successful with his experiments, treating cretinism with iodine and syphilis with malarial fever.

> The recipe for Scrambled Jaureggs comes, I think, from the "febrile bout" that takes place during a malarial cure. The pan is so hot it is almost burning up. The butter browns, the beaten eggs, seasoned with red pepper, go in and out so fast they are slightly streaky with the brownish butter.
> And do not worry that butter and eggs are an unhealthy combination. Would you rather have malaria?

NOTE

"my name was not even to be commemorated . . ."; Josef and Renée Gicklhorn, *Sigmund Freuds akademische Laufbahn* (Vienna: Urban & Schwarzenberg, 1960), pp. 53–57.

LOMBROSO'S CAESAR SALAD

Cesare Lombroso, an Italian Jew, found his path to international psychiatric fame by investigating the links between genius and insanity. He could not stop there but went on with genius and criminality, genius and degeneration, genius and anatomy—yet the man could not tell the difference between epilepsy and hysteria. A "phantast" I called him, but his final work, on the relationship of genius with salad, remains valuable, as the present example, named for him, attests.

> Rub salad bowl with garlic. In bowl, place pieces of lettuce, chicory, escarole, or other greens. Pour 1/4 cup olive oil over the greens and toss lightly. Mix 2 tbs. lemon juice and 2 tbs. good red wine and pour

over the greens. Add a handful of croutons, salt and pepper to taste, and toss again.

NOTE

"A phantast . . ."; letter to Stefan Zweig, 19 October 1920.

CARL KOLLER'S CARP

We always used to say around medical school: patients, like fish, should be judged by the eye. When buying a fish, you must look it in the eye (do not do this, of course, for frozen fish or breaded fish cutlets). It is easier with fish than with patients, who must be kept behind you on the couch. Yet only the eye reveals the degree of freshness. This I learned from Carl Koller, an old friend from medical school days and a great ophthalmologist. We were standing around once, experimenting with cocaine, which Carl adapted as an anaesthetic for eye surgery (thereby achieving fame), when he said, "Do you look your fish in the eye, Sigi?" I had to admit that I did not.

The white eye of the boiled carp should not be removed. Most *Feinschmeckers* prefer it to the empty socket. Koller even preferred to draw attention to it, by burying the fish, except for its eye, in this German beer sauce.

Sauté a few diced carrots, onions, and celery. Stir in 2 tbs. flour. Add a glass of beer, 2 tbs. vinegar, the juice of half a lemon with its grated rind, and 1 tbs. brown sugar. Cook until the sauce begins to thicken. Place carp in a buttered baking dish and pour sauce over the whole fish except for the eye. If you want to call attention to the eye, make circles radiating from it with slivered almonds, and bake in a 350° oven for about 15 minutes or until done.

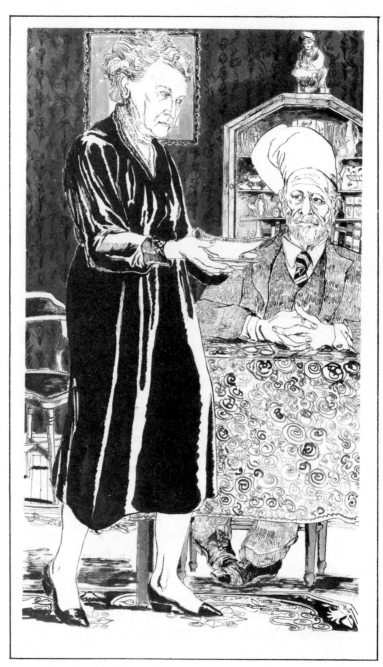

Martha's Bernays Sauce

II.

MARRIAGE AND FAMILY

With Two Kinds of Bernays Sauce

"Now it occurs to me that we would need two or three little rooms to live and eat in and to receive a guest and a stove in which the fire for our meals never goes out."

—Letter to Martha, 18 August 1882,
in *Letters of Sigmund Freud,*
1873–1939, ed. E. L. Freud

It is the privilege of age to correct the follies of youth—
even one's own. Years ago I discovered that children's fantasies interpreting their parents' intercourse as a sadistic
act determined the course of their future neuroses. These
primal fantasies, as I termed them, circling about the dis-
appearance of parents and the subsequent whispers and
strangulated moans from behind closed doors, could so delay dinner, burn the roast, or let the soup get cold, that a
child's instinctual gratifications could suffer nearly irreversible damage.

The correction I am now able to bring after decades of
silent attention to the fantasies of my patients is not directed at the primal fantasies themselves. The core of the
theory has been confirmed in case after case: neurotics suffer from reminiscences. But the focus of this suffering is
not, as I thought then, the bed. It is the table! It is not the
imagined sadism of the primal scene that harms the child,
but the actual sadism of the primal meal.

These reminiscences are usually covered by screen
memories of the family romance: the little loving clan
gathered around the table, smiling mother spooning warm
Knödels, bearded father bowed in grace, the children gig-
gling, little kicks and pinches between the chairs, perhaps
some *Schmarotzer* of a dear impoverished uncle making
jokes.

Then, as the analysis proceeds, the truth is laid bare.
The repressed reminiscence returns: one sits again, three
years old face-to-face with strained spinach and mashed
meat congealing on the plate under the brutal command:
"Stop playing around and eat!" The crucial factor here is
that of distancing. The small child has no distance between
his face and the food: his head is barely six inches from his
plate. The sadistic torture of this position is made all the

worse by parents with long necks and long arms who ignore the injustice of the child's inferior size. All the while the child is told that only if one eats can one grow.

We thus see how the imagined sadism of the bedroom—that the parents may be murdering each other—is actually a wish to escape from the terror of the primal meal, and the desire to watch big people in the bedroom actually a conversion of the memory of being watched by big people at the table.

Of the various neurotic symptoms that can be traced back to the primal meal, none is more devastating than carrot envy. The child staring into his soup fixes his or her gaze on a piece of carrot submerged there. "Must I eat that, all of that? It is so big!"

He or she then looks into the soups of siblings, rivalrously discovering that they have what seems a smaller carrot, or better yet, none at all. Intense carrot envy ensues, which emerges in adolescence as a curiosity about all carrot-shaped objects, their size and length—and absence.

But let us return to the primal meal itself and the command: "Stop playing around and eat!"

Here are sown the seeds for that long-lasting opposition between playing around and eating. *Essen ohne Freud,* we call it, a joylessness in food; for playing around has become the alternative to a good dinner. Don Juanism, coupled with the fast-food habit (*consummatio rapida*), can be expected as a consequence.

(This condition, I am told by Minna, is witnessed in modern cinema, where it is the fashion for the flirtatious heroine in restaurant scenes to toy with her food, and for the conquering hero never to pause to see what is in the icebox or make himself a little sandwich. I do not favor the cinema myself; not only because there is never enough time to get there with all that we have to do for dinner, but because when one has seen as many screen memories as I have, who needs celluloid?)

MARTHA'S RING CAKE

Food and Martha!—old I am, stoic my nature, the events now so faint in memory, yet how I still dwell upon the early scenes of our first encounters. Food played the *Schadchen,* the go-between, in our love. Her first gift to me was a cake she had baked herself; her first sign of physical affection took place under our family dining table, when she pressed my hand in gratitude for my having taken her place card with her name on it as souvenir of this first meal together. And that time when the ring she had given me sprang apart, dropping its pearl, and I surreptitiously supposed she had at that moment suffered a change of feelings toward me, it so turned out that she was in fact enjoying a slice of cake (a *Gugelhupf*). Even that first sight of her, that indelibly enduring image which drove me wild, was of Martha seated at table, peeling an apple.

> Butter a ring mold. In the bottom of the mold, arrange a layer of thinly sliced apples (peeled and soaked for a few minutes in a little lemon juice and rum). Make a batter combining 2 cups flour, 1/2 tsp. salt, 1/3 cup sugar, 2 tsp. baking powder, 2 tsp. grated orange peel, 1/2 tsp. vanilla extract, 1/3 cup butter, 1 egg, and 1/2 cup milk. When batter is smooth, add 1/2 cup raisins. Pour batter over apple layer. Bake in 375° oven for about 30 minutes. Turn it out on a cake rack to cool and dust with confectioner's sugar.

OUR ANNIVERSARY HAM

Ernest Jones was the only person later on allowed by my family to read the voluminous love letters I sent Martha (at least one a day during four years of courtship). Since his biography has revealed so much of my life at that time, describing, as he so romantically puts it, "the volcano within" me, I do not think I am revealing anything indiscreet to give the following recipe here. It stemmed from my intense aversion to Martha's family (particularly her most obstinate mother), with their superstitious orthodox ways. "They would have preferred you to marry an old Rabbi or *Schochet,*" I wrote Martha, which particularly amused her because a *Schochet* is a butcher who follows kosher rules, and her family dining was kosher if ever anyone's was. I tried hard to win her away from such food restrictions, although, as Jones found worthy to point out, it took a long time to get her to like ham. Yet, this dish converted her, and we never failed to have it on our anniversary. Ever after, guests about to be served this at our table would lift their eyes in astonishment. But I, as house *Schochet,* just dug in.

> Sprinkle a little brown sugar over the ham, which you
> must score in some design of other (diamonds are
> always appropriate). Put ham in a roasting pan and
> pour a cup of champagne around it (proceed to drink
> the rest of the bottle while waiting for the ham to
> cook). Bake in 375° oven for about 20 minutes per
> pound. The champagne sauce alone will make you
> forget your kosher mother-in-law.

NOTES
"the volcano within"; Jones, *Life and Work,* vol. 1, p. 138.
"They would have preferred you"; ibid., p. 134.

MARTHA'S BERNAYS SAUCE

A Bernays does not yield its secret to the slapdash temperament (I have learned that if I have learned anything!). As Martha used to say, "In our house no one speaks of nerves"—and she lived to be ninety.

Be sure the ingredients for the sauce are first laid out carefully in Martha's style. She laid out my clothes, chose my linens, socks, and handkerchiefs, even put the toothpaste on my toothbrush. Small and delicate as she was, she ran our household and, with a big wicker basket over her arm, did the marketing.

> Boil down 2 tbs. chopped shallots, and $\frac{1}{2}$ cup tarragon vinegar, until only a few tbs. of liquid remain. Put this, with 2 tsp. lemon juice, in top of Double-Bleuler, over low flame. Add spoon of cold water. Slowly add 4 oz. melted butter and 4 beaten egg yolks (see "An Egg Is Being Beaten" but not at this moment which is crucial), whisking constantly until sauce thickens. Remove from heat immediately, add salt and pepper, and 1 tsp. of fresh chopped tarragon.

NOTE
"She laid out my clothes . . ."; Paul Roazen, *Brother Animal, the Story of Freud and Tausk* (Middlesex: Penguin, 1973), p. 39; Jones, *Life and Work,* vol. 1, pp. 116–19; A. Kardiner, *My Analysis with Freud* (New York, Norton, 1977), p. 19.

MINNA'S BERNAYS SAUCE

My sister Anna married Eli Bernays. My nephew in New York was the publisher Edward Bernays. And there was Emmeline, my mother-in-law, who put Bernays on Hamburger (being a Hamburger herself, from Wandsbek). Any way you pour it, eating with the in-laws meant Bernays.

As Martha and Minna were sisters, so is this second Bernays sauce kin to the first. It is, I confess, the more stalwart and astringent of the two (instead of the $1/2$ cup of tarragon vinegar, use $1/4$ cup white wine and $1/4$ cup white vinegar, a touch more tarragon, a suggestion of red pepper, and brighten everything by the supplement of an unconscious tomato (see "Unconscious Tomatoes") which you have pureed to a paste.

In regard to the tomato, it is my duty to deny the gossip that persists to this day that Minna, my sister-in-law, who came to live with us in 1896, and stayed to the end, had any liaison with me other than as companion in the curiosity of the mind and the mouth. The joys of walking tours around Salzburg, of traveling together in Italy, of tasting foreign dishes—this I admit willingly. (Martha could not get packed quickly and she suffered from gastric disturbances.) And yet, what use denial? There are so many "Freudians" out there who will only call this an unconscious means of affirmation. You can't win.

MINNA'S MEATLOAF

Chop an onion, a celery stalk, and a green pepper, and combine with ¹/₂ lb. ground beef, ¹/₂ lb. ground veal, 1 egg, dash horseradish, 1 tsp. paprika, salt, pepper, and 1 chopped Unconscious Tomato (see "Unconscious Tomatoes"). Mold into loaf. Place in a greased loaf pan. Bake at 350° for 1 hour.

STRONE

This thick soup of the Austro-Hungarian Empire was a specialty of my sister-in-law.

In a thick kettle, she browned several ounces of good sliced sausage in a few tbs. of olive oil. She added 3 pints of good beef stock and this was brought to the boil. Then she chopped up a wonderful variety of vegetables and added them to the pot, including, usually, a handful of green beans, a handful of white beans, several stalks of chopped celery, a small shredded red cabbage, 2 sliced onions, a few chopped tomatoes, a cup of fresh peas, several leaves of roughly torn spinach, plenty of chopped parsley, a clove of minced garlic, and a few tbs. of rice. She seasoned all this with a *bouquet garni,* salt and pepper, and 1 tsp. of paprika. After the Strone simmers for a few hours, Austrians like to serve it with a grating of Sbrinz cheese, but in our house Parmesan was always the choice on Minna's Strone.

ROAST BIRDS À LA LOVRANA

One summer I took Martha and the children to Lovrana, a small fishing village on the Adriatic. We stayed at a comfortable hotel, where, since my brother Alexander and I used to enjoy the warm salt water so much that we often refused to swim to shore even for lunch, that very obliging establishment would have a waiter wade out to us, balancing adroitly a tray of refreshments, usually little roast birds on toast, and sometimes even cigars and matches. The reader may no longer remember what first-class accommodations were like before the Great War and may find it hard to imagine such service. You need not imagine what eating little birds was like, for I obtained the hotel's recipe.

> Drawn, washed, and basted in olive oil, then seasoned with coarse salt, pepper, and a sprig of fresh rosemary inserted under the skin, they were baked in a shallow pan in a 425° oven for about 20 minutes, then served on toast with a little currant jelly. I recommend them to all but the English, who seem so squeamish, if not hysterical, when it comes to eating their all-too-abundant sparrows and wrens. (Ernest Jones, though he had a taste for little birds—see "Welsh Omelette"—would have been aghast at the prospect of roasting them, and so I never told him this story.)

NOTE
Cf. Martin Freud, *Sigmund Freud, Man and Father*, pp. 45–46.

DISPLACEMATS

"Where would we be without conventions?" They keep our lives in order and form the foundations of regular marriage, family, and social life. I did not myself engage in marriage or family counseling, nor would I be—perish the thought—what they call today a certified family counselor. After all, I was up to my beard in it, with Martha there, and Minna living with us, and my mother staying alive to ninety-five, and six children. I did, however, analyze my daughter Anna, thereby saving her from the possibilities of a bad marriage, or any marriage for that matter.

Nonetheless, I learned from my patients many things about the conventions that maintain families, like regular meal hours and habitual place settings at the table. Place settings are particularly important, whether for each person or for the main dishes set before father or mother for serving.

But custom stales. Foreknowledge disturbs forepleasure. One seductive attraction of the restaurant—see "Eating Out"—is precisely that we do not know where we shall be placed, thereby stimulating the unconscious to excite us with frissons of disorientation: Where did I put my coat? Which way was the men's room? Is that a mirror, or another room over there?

To provide equivalently fertile disorientation in the all-too-familiar home, I have discovered the displacemat, taking the idea directly from the dream. There we find fear of one object (the mother's sharp temper) to be displaced onto another object (the sharp teeth of a snarling dog). In other cases, emotion itself may be displaced: I dare not desire my father's chocolate éclair, so I hate all éclairs, or I desire an éclair surrogate, his hat (whence comes the displaced phrase, "I'll eat my hat"—of course meaning my father).

To cure the boredom of family meals, therefore, use displacemats. Put the soup tureen down right in front of your little son. Put his plate on its displacemat in the middle of the table. Set the lazy susan, replete with catsup and toothpicks, on father's displacemat, in front of him. Before the guest, place a large pewter dish of gourds or a grape display with candles, or the bowl of glads. Make him guess and have to ask where his plate and displacemat are. Sit six on one side of the table and none on the other. Or serve your elaborately home-cooked meal in sectioned aluminum dinner trays. These are the best displacemats of all, but care and discretion must be exercised in this case lest you displace the family itself and they all disperse to the television set, or, worse, they start the neurotic habit of eating out (see "Eating Out").

NOTE

"Where would we be . . ."; Joseph Wortis, *Fragments of an Analysis with Freud* (New York: McGraw-Hill, 1975), p. 104.

BERGGASSE BEANS WITH BACON
(*Bohnen mit Speck*)

Part of our apartment, Berggasse 19, was situated just above Kornmehl's Butcher Shop. (Indeed, after the other children moved out, my daughter Anna occupied for herself and her practice the two front rooms directly over that meat market.) As my patients will attest, on the way to and from analysis, they had to pass the display windows, such superb witness to the harmony of Eros and Thanatos: meats from slaughtered animals dressed and cured by loving hands—*Tafelspitz, Rostbraten, Geselchtes, Kalbsschnitzel mit Nieren, Lungenbraten,* and *Sulz* (or what is in English so unpleasantly called "head cheese") still bearing its remnants of hog bristles—all these for the patient to enjoy as he turned into the doorway and mounted the stairs for his hour. Sometimes, during the earlier years of my practice, I would instruct the more composed patients to stop at the deli counter on the way up and bring me some *Bohnen mit Speck,* a good snack during those long analytical sessions, and cheap too.

> Boil ¼ lb. diced bacon until tender. Add 1 lb. broad beans, pepper, a few tbs. of chopped onion and carrot, and ½ tsp. caraway seeds. Cook until beans are tender. Thicken liquid with arrowroot, and serve in a deli container.

NOTE
Cf. Edmund Engleman, *Berggasse 19, Sigmund Freud's House and Offices, Vienna 1938* (New York: Basic Books, 1976).

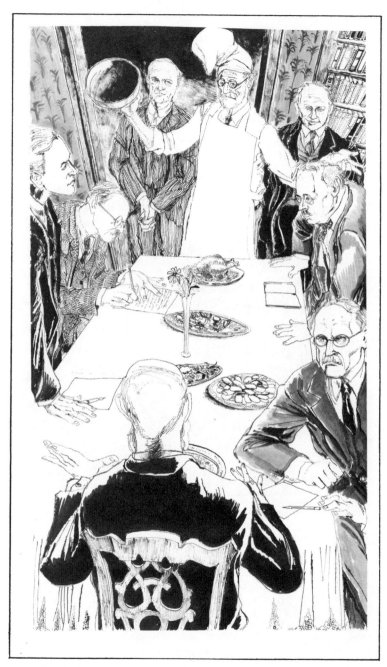

Table d'hote

III.

FRENCH COOKING

Including Charcot-Broiling, Bernheim's Suggestions, and Duck Liver *Hystérique*

"And on top of that the wretched megalomania of the French for insisting on 4¹/₂ hours of theatre as they do on 5 or 6 course meals. To enjoy one's way through something quickly, allowing interest to help conquer fatigue, is too plebeian for them; so they prolong a 2¹/₂ hour play by 2 hours of entr'acte during which one can, it's true, go out into the beautiful evening and drink beer, smoke a cigar and eat oranges; but if one returns too early (as one invariably does), one suffers the ghastly tortures of anticipation in the oven."

—Letter to Martha, 8 November 1885,
in *Letters of Sigmund Freud,
1873–1939*, ed. E. L. Freud

CHARCOT-BROILED LAMB CHOPS

Jean Martin Charcot, my great teacher at the Salpêtrière in Paris, who took the first step in elucidating hysteria, also introduced me to lamb chops done this way.

> He would truly hypnotize the lamb chops in a marinade (puree a handful of rosemary—the herb of memory—with 2 cloves of mashed garlic, and a little olive oil). They would stand motionless in this marinade throughout his lecture. When the lecture was finished (usually 2 to 4 hours), the chops were broiled on a grill over his Bunsen burner (but an outdoor Charcot-grill is just as good and keeps the smoke out of your lecture hall). Cooked just rare, the chops were served with a topping of rosemary butter to wake them up (a few tbs. butter, rosemary, and mashed garlic beaten together in a bowl until blended, then chilled).

As I wrote after his death in 1893, "As a teacher Charcot was perfectly fascinating: each of his lectures was a little masterpiece in construction and composition, perfect in style, and so impressive that the words spoken echoed in one's ears, and the subject demonstrated remained before one's eyes for the rest of the day." The garlic on his lamb chops stays with you all day too.

CHARCOT-BROILING

Nowadays, there are iron grills for the top of the stove, electric broilers built into ovens, cookouts with special woods, mesquite, white oak, hickory, and other transatlantic imports. But nothing compares with the old-fashioned Charcot-Broiler for giving that taste of true French elegance.

Paris was where I first encountered this type of cooking. Indeed, it is where I first really began cooking at all. In exile from "my little Princess" (as I used to call Martha before we got married), without an easy command of French, in penury and reduced to bread, beer, and that French coffee, I was enormously indebted to Jean Martin Charcot, the most famous neurologist of the day and the inventor of the method of broiling that still bears his name, for taking me into his circle of gourmets. I named my son Martin after him, and in tribute to all that he taught me about cuisine I should even dedicate this book to him, so much did he mean to me. To face the Master in his own home at a white-tie, white-glove dinner, I sturdied myself with a small dose of cocaine and shot through the evening without a blunder. Charcot complimented me, saying I had fattened up (*engraissé*) since being with him, but at the dinner, as I wrote later, "we were not given very much to eat." Strange, because he charged exorbitantly high fees.

I did, however, meet many important and curious people at those Charcot dinners, including his buxom twenty-year-old daughter, who on one occasion wore a Greek costume and never spoke a word to me. She may have been suffering from a globus hystericus or a paralysis, since it was not all that easy for Charcot to separate his home life from the office. Toward midnight we went back to the dining room for a little more to eat and lots to drink. I took a cup of chocolate. But, "It was so boring," I noted, "I nearly burst; only the bit of cocaine prevented me from doing so."

No, I do not think I will dedicate my cookbook to him; a son was enough.

NOTE

Cf. Letters of Sigmund Freud, 92, 94, 96.

BERNHEIM'S SUGGESTIONS

In the summer of 1889, while still a young doctor, and in the hope of perfecting my hypnotic technique, I journeyed to Nancy, France, and spent several weeks as a spectator of Dr. Hippolyte Bernheim's astonishing experiments upon his hospital patients. It was there that, spellbound, I received the profound impression that powerful mental processes lay hidden from the consciousness of man.

Bernheim put people into trances and then made suggestions to them so that when they came to, they would no longer suffer their debilitating symptoms, such as loss of appetite or indigestion. Sometimes it worked, sometimes it did not, and there was a beautiful indifference—*la belle indifférence,* as the French called it—regarding results.

It was a happy time in Bernheim's clinic—all those people walking around in trances, in the corridors, out in the gardens, doing this and that, and no one afterward recalling anything about it. Sometimes they missed their meals by unfortunately not coming to in time. Bernheim, too, did not remember much; come to think of it now, I do not remember much of what I learned there either.

I had brought along to Nancy one of my own patients, a woman of good birth, who had been handed over to me because no one knew what to do with her. It is not that I thought trips to France would improve her highly gifted hysteria; it was because she had always relapsed after my own attempts at hypnotic influence on her misery.

After seating her comfortably and quietly at his dining table, Bernheim brought out an appetizer course of salmon, ham, or some other dish, each one a fine example of French cuisine. My patient would calmly consume the appetizer, with Bernheim merely making polite conversation with her during this time. Then a salad course was served, with yet more casual conversation. Finally, after about an hour, the main course was presented, and it would always be the same as the appetizer, except on a large platter and prepared in a grander way. Salmon mousse, for example, was the appetizer on the first day, and the main course was a minted salmon. On the second day, the appetizer was duck liver, followed by a main course of roast duck. On the third day, it was a *jambon en croûte* followed by a large baked ham.

Each time the main course was brought out, my patient said to Bernheim:

—Didn't we just have this?

He would reply, simply:

—Did we?

—Yes, she would go on, I'm almost certain we've had this before.

—Tell me about it, he would say, and there usually followed a long recollection of the appetizer course, along with many other things.

Unfortunately, the patient proceeded to become only more hysterical as the days, and meals, went on. Bernheim's suggestion method had great value, I did not doubt, and I continued to use it myself for a while in my Vienna practice, with my own modifications, suggesting to my patients, after putting them in hypnotic states, various behaviors to cure their malaise: try sardines on toast; use starched and large damask napkins; go to the Belle Vue restaurant and order their *Milchrahmstrudel* and a *Kaffe mit Schlag*. But after eighteen months of this imported French foolishness, I had had enough, even though some of the patients prospered, gaining weight and going into a trance smiling and expectant.

I soon moved on to the "free association" method, in which the main course usually bore only a slight resemblance or hint of the appetizer, if that, and usually came as a complete surprise to all concerned.

Nonetheless, the reader may wish to experiment with Bernheim's Suggestions, so I give the first three.

NOTE

"I had brought along to Nancy . . ."; Jones, *Life and Work,* vol. 1, p. 238.

I.

THE SALMON MOUSSE AT NANCY

Dissolve an envelope of unflavored gelatin in a cup of boiling water. Let cool. Stir in 1/2 cup mayonnaise, 2 tbs. sherry, 1/4 cup finely chopped cashews or other nuts, and a bare suggestion of chopped dill. Add 2 cups flaked poached or canned salmon, and 1 cup firmly whipped cream. Pour into a salmon mold, so that the patient can clearly see it is a fish, and refrigerate for several hours. Serve with crackers. (Main course must also be salmon, such as "The Salmon at Nancy.")

THE SALMON AT NANCY

Place a salmon steak over some chopped shallots in a buttered baking dish. Add 1/4 cup vinegar. Dot with mint butter (chopped mint and butter mixed in palm of hand). Broil in 300° oven for about 15 minutes, or until done, basting frequently. Serve topped with more mint butter and a sprig of fresh mint.

II.

JAMBON EN CROÛTE AT NANCY

Bernheim was in a hurry so he did not bother to make puff pastries for these canapés. Instead he used thin slices of French bread. Place a slice of baked ham on the bread and top with a little Mornay Sauce. Top the canapé with more grated Gruyère. Toast briefly under broiler. (Main course must also be ham, such as "The Ham at Nancy.")

BERNHEIM'S MORNAY SAUCE

Stir 4 tbs. butter and 4 tbs. flour smooth over medium heat. Slowly add 1½ cups milk and continue to stir over heat till creamy. Add 1 cup chicken stock, ½ cup grated Gruyère cheese, and ⅓ cup grated Parmesan. Stir again over low heat until cheese is melted. Salt and pepper to taste.

THE HAM AT NANCY

Marinate overnight a small ham (3 lbs.) in a baking dish with a large glass of white wine, a few sautéed carrots and onions, parsley, minced garlic, bay leaf, and a few cloves. Next day, simmer everything for 1½ hours in 325° oven, basting frequently. Sauté more vegetables (a little lettuce, onions, carrots, beans, and peas) to surround the ham. Spoon sauce over everything and serve.

III.

DUCK LIVER *HYSTÉRIQUE*

Simmer one large duck liver (per person) in water for
15 minutes. In food processor, puree the cooked liver
with 1 small peeled and seeded tomato, a few tbs.
butter, 1 tbs. cognac, and salt and pepper. Chill for
several hours and serve on toast points. (Main course
must also be duck, such as "The Duck at Nancy.")

THE DUCK AT NANCY

Roast a 3-lb. duckling in 375° oven for an hour.
Meanwhile, in a saucepan of water, boil 1 lb. of green
peas and several small white onions for about a
minute. Drain. Pour off fat from cooked duckling and
surround the duck with the vegetables. In saucepan,
quickly boil 3 tbs. mint jelly with 2 tbs. sherry
vinegar. Pour this over the duck and vegetables.
Season with salt and pepper and return everything to
the oven for a few more minutes.

BRAISED OX TONGUE WITH APHASIA SAUCE

I was fascinated by language and words long before I began
to notice the slips of the tongue in everyday life and the curious plays of words in dreams and jokes. In fact, my first
major book was on speech disorders, the aphasias. Though
it was a fine piece of anatomical research, it took nine years
to dispose of 257 copies. What does that matter now? It
yielded this recipe for tongue that I have kept on enjoying
long after the anatomy of its function is lost beyond recall.

Simmer the tongue with some chopped onions, mushrooms, celery, and carrots, a glass of red wine, a spoonful of currants, 2 tbs. red wine vinegar, a dash of G. Stanley Hall's Worcester Sauce, a bay leaf, and enough water to cover. After a few hours, the tip of the tongue should be tender. Skin it. Remove bay leaf, and puree the vegetables in a food processor, adding salt and pepper to taste. Pamper the tongue with the puree.

SLIPS OF THE TONGUE IN MADEIRA SAUCE

My essay on the little errors we all make in everyday life soon proved the most popular. It took no time at all until a momentary lapse in speaking—forgetting a name, mispronouncing a word, getting the syllables backwards—came to be called "a Freudian slip." The explanation that I first gave still holds for these faulty and chance actions. A *lapsus lingua* expresses unconscious wishes in a condensed, distorted, and disguised form. But this earlier explanation, though necessary, is insufficient. We must push the inquiry yet further, asking why does the repressed return via the tongue? Why does one feel shame when forced to "eat" words one has regretted saying? Why this specific "organ choice" (as Adler might say in his vulgar language)? Is it not the unsatisfied need of the organ, a tongue that has unfulfilled requirements for tastiness that becomes obliged to call attention to itself by symptomatic means—malapropisms, misplaced consonants, or refusal to come up with the word on its very tip—that claims immediate attention to its need for satisfactions beyond words? The cure becomes evident: eat first, talk later.

Boil the tongue until tender (about 1 hour) in lightly salted water. Meanwhile, sauté a handful of fresh

mushrooms in butter and oil, with a tbs. of chopped
onions or shallots. Add 1 cup of the water in which
the tongue has been boiling and 1 tbs. tomato paste.
Boil for several minutes until reduced to a few tbs.
Add a glass of madeira with a tbs. of arrowroot stirred
in. Boil until sauce thickens. When tongue is tender,
remove the skin and cut into slips of about 2 inches
each. Add to Madeira sauce. Correct seasoning with
salt and pepper and serve topped with parsley.

THE LOWERING OF THE LENTIL LEVEL

The lentil is not your common bean. Its lovely flatness, its
dull ochre or pink, or the yellow *dal* of India, and the way
lentils both give and borrow flavors all demand from the
cook the greatest respect. Soaking them in water with
some cut up old sausage and stewing them into a soup until the level drops and the mess condenses—Janet's way—
is not enough. Worse: it can make you hysterical. In fact,
Janet invented the term *abaissement du niveau mental*
and ascribed to this lowering of the lentil level all the fran-
tic symptoms of his women cases. But Janet did not know
beans about lentils, or about hysterics either. I soon figured out that their trouble had to do with the saltpeter that
was being put in their food at the Salpêtrière hospital. I
took my discovery back to Vienna. The rest is history.

Janet and I kept up a "guerrilla war" for much of our
lives because he was always out to steal my recipes all the
while accusing me of purloining his. That man belonged in
a lentil institution.

NOTE
"guerrilla war"; Clark, *Freud,* p. 93.

VEAL NEURASTHENIA

Already in the early 1890s I described the symptoms of neurasthenia—pressure in the head, exhaustion, digestive disturbances accompanied by flatus and constipation, back pain and sexual weakness. Next I detached these symptoms from the more fundamental problem of anxiety, or anxiety neurosis. Quite a step, if I say so myself. In time I came to understand that neurasthenia is not a nervous disorder, not even a weakness of nerves, but a failure of nerve.

In the language of Adler and Rank, it is a problem of the Will, or as they used to pronounce it, the "Veal." The neurasthenic patient, after all, is a kind of *vitellone* or *Kalb,* usually mooning through his first calf-love.

I say "his" deliberately because, as I have always maintained, "girls are normally healthy and not neurasthenic." On physical examination, the neurasthenic's flesh proves to be moist, tender, and pale, very much in fact like the whitish-pink of good veal. The eyes are unusually soft and dilated.

The neurasthenic tends to keep himself penned up in his room or mopes around the local dairy bar eating quarts of ice cream. The treatment of choice in such cases is usually tonics for the will. Yet, though the patient is usually docile and cooperative, such cases show slow improvement, because, as a rule, though the veal is willing, the flesh is simply too weak. Veal Neurasthenia, therefore, is my own unfailing remedy for such *schlemiels.* Care must be taken that it not be overcooked. It should even be a little tough; in fact, the tougher, the better.

Take a nice (3 or 4 lb.) rump of veal and have your butcher tie it up tight. Let it stand in this condition for a few hours before roasting. Coat the roast in a mixture of 2 tbs. flour, 1 tsp. chili powder, 1 tsp.

paprika, and salt and pepper. Roast in 350° oven for $1/2$ hour, basting occasionally with a little melted butter. Meanwhile, simmer a cup of brown stock with $1/2$ cup cognac, until it is reduced by a third.

Continue roasting the veal for another half hour, this time basting with the stock-cognac mixture. Sautéed onions or other hearty vegetables may be added to the pan, but do not worry about the decoration of the dish. It is the meat that counts, and for once it must not be tender.

NOTE
"girls are normally healthy"; *Letters to Wilhelm Fliess,* p. 69.

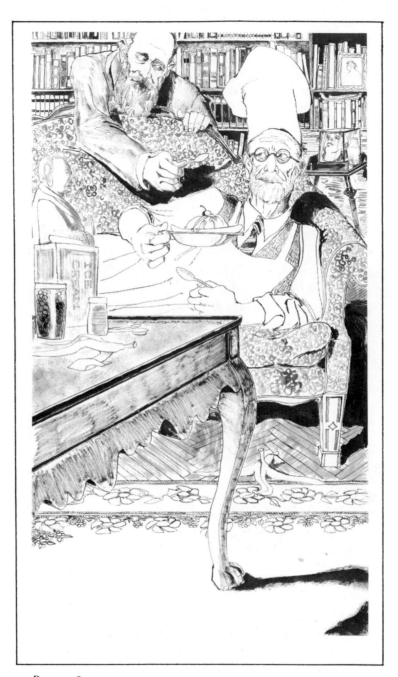

Banana O.

IV.

DISHES FROM THE MASTER CHEFS

Josef's Breuered Beef, Split Fliess Soup, Kraepelin Suzettes, et al.

"They must all cook at our fire."
—Freud quoted in "Profile,
Dr. Ernest Jones," *The Observer*
(London), 26 July 1953

It quickly became clear to me that my neurotic patients' anxiety had much to do with eating habits; and in particular it struck me how inevitably Luncheon Interruptus practiced by a man or woman led to anxiety neurosis.

Luncheon Interruptus occurs in several ways: the most commonly used method is the telephone, timed to ring only minutes or even seconds after one sits down to lunch. It is almost always effective. Another device is the lunchtime visitor who will knock on the door just after luncheon has commenced. This is often less effective than the telephone since one must usually ask the uninvited guest to join in the meal; one then has a luncheon à trois.

At first I thought there might only be two occasions for anxiety in Luncheon Interruptus: in the woman, a fear of becoming fat, and in the man, a fear that his appetite might fail.

But then I found convincing evidence in a number of cases that anxiety neurosis also appeared where there was no question of these two factors being present, where it was really of no importance to the people concerned whether they finished lunch or not. Thus anxiety neurosis could not be a prolongation of recollected, hysterical anxiety. Its source was not to be looked for in psychical events. What generates anxiety must be some physical factor in eating itself. But what can this factor be?

To resolve this question I collected all the conditions under which I found anxiety arising from culinary causes. They seemed at first a most heterogeneous collection:

I. Anxiety occurring in virginal subjects (people who have not yet eaten a truly good meal, and do not know what one tastes like, although they have heard about good food or seen one of those rare movies where the actors dine well). Numerous instances of this have been confirmed, in both sexes, though principally in women.

II. Anxiety occurring in subjects who are deliberately abstinent—prudes (a neuropathic type). These are men and women characterized by pedantry, xenophobia, or a love of cleanliness, who regard anything gourmand as a foreign abomination. They content themselves with the consumption of raw carrots, a hard-boiled egg, or anything that is deliberately anti-gourmet in its preparation.

III. Anxiety in subjects who are abstinent from necessity: women who are destitute or who are neglected by their husbands or who cannot be satisfied owing to their husbands' general lack of resources. This form of anxiety neurosis can certainly be acquired.

IV. Anxiety in women who are subject to Luncheon Interruptus against their will, usually after they have prepared some very tempting cuisine, or (what is very similar) in women whose husbands suffer from jockulatio praecox (the chronic need to watch football games or other sporting events in lieu of fine dining).

V. Anxiety in men who practice Luncheon Interruptus, and still more in men who excite their appetites in various ways with dips, martinis, and other so-called appetizers, but do not then employ their stimulated taste buds in going on to the main course.

VI. Anxiety in men who force themselves to lick their plate clean though it is beyond their desire or strength.

VII. Anxiety in men who are abstinent from contingent circumstances: in young men, for example, married to women older than themselves, with whom they are suddenly disgusted or reminded too much of their mothers; or in neurasthenics who have been diverted from lunch by intellectual occupations without compensating for this by snacking; or in men whose appetite is beginning to decline and who abstain from lunch in marriage on account of unpleasant sensations post luncheon. *Post prandium omne animal triste est.*

How are all these different instances to be combined? The factor of abstinence is the most frequently recurring one. If we bear in mind our observation that anxiety occurs after Luncheon Interruptus even in those who are anaesthetic and used to eating crappy food (see "Jung Food"), we may lay it down that what we are dealing with is simply a physical accumulation of hunger tension. The accumulation is due to discharge being held up. Anxiety neurosis from Luncheon Interruptus is thus like hysteria, a neurosis due to dammed-up excitation, to a desire to eat those tomatoes or hunks of meat but with a failure to eat them once served.

Needless to say, I can no longer recommend Luncheon Interruptus as a method for weight control.

KRAFFT-EBING LADY'S SLIPPERS

This seductive little sweet was stolen from that famous author of perverse erotica, Professor Richard von Krafft-Ebing, whose *Psychopathia Sexualis* was to be found on the nightstand by the bed of everyone of my generation. Krafft-Ebing's work was the first modern volume of medically authenticated pornography. It was published in 1886 when the Professor, then age forty-six, was finding his own strength ebbing. Rapists, stranglers, necrophiliacs; *frotteurs* and flagellants; defilers of statues and despoilers of children; *renifleurs* and *stercoraires*—all parade through its pages, but not a single recipe for anything to eat. Even in the cases of fetishism not one food is mentioned, yet who does not know the state of secret excitation brought on at night by the anticipation of chocolates criminally hidden under the pillow?

His book today seems so old-fashioned. It is not even a good bedside companion; personally, I prefer to take cookbooks to bed.

Although K.E. (as he was called in the leather bars) and I were in Vienna together, we shared little. He never referred one recipe to me. Only when a former case of his came later to me for treatment and told me how K.E. had tried, unsuccessfully, to divert his shoe fetish into the substitute pleasure of this dessert, did I purloin the formula. But Krafft-Ebing understood nothing of sublimation, and nothing of desserts either. A good dessert is sublime, not a sublimation.

Pour 1 cup of warm milk (to remind one of bedtime) over $1/4$ lb. of stale ladyfingers (a necrophilic thought in itself). Pour into food processor, with 3 eggs, $1/8$ cup sugar, 1 tbs. raisins, and a few tbs. of fig liqueur. Panting, turn processor on and off several times.

The mold, in the shape of a lady's slipper, is admittedly hard to find, although some of the more exotic kitchen supply stores may still stock them. I am told that K.E. also had molds in the shape of bloomers and rubber raincoats, but I have never seen these myself, nor do I think they are necessary.

Butter the mold and sprinkle lightly with sugar. Fill with batter and bake in 325° oven for $1/2$ hour, or until it, and you, are set. Unmold, and serve slippers decorated with a single dried fig, among other things.

JOSEF'S BREUERED BEEF

Breuer still does not receive enough credit for this all too commonplace dish which the public somehow thinks I invented; it was, however, the true reason for the break-up of our great and productive friendship.

His patient, the now world-famous Anna O., whose classic hysteria taught us all so much, told Breuer her terrifying fantasies and hallucinations, including the details of the first appearances of her extraordinary hysterical symptoms: paralysis of three limbs, talking gibberish or only English, *tussis nervosa* (coughing fits), blurred vision, and especially, not eating. No sooner were the details of the symptoms told than they were cured. It was Anna O. who thus called this new procedure—psychoanalysis—"the talking cure."

She was twenty-one, of lively mind, and fascinating. Poor Breuer developed a strong countertransference to his Fräulein Anna (see "Banana O"). He tried to break off the talks; not, however, before Anna O. was to go into a hysterical childbirth based no doubt on a phantom pregnancy she had developed in response to her devoted analyst. Shocked, and in a cold sweat, Breuer fled the scene and next day left with his wife for a second honeymoon in Venice, resulting in a new daughter in the Breuer family.

Ah, hysterics—Katerina, Elisabeth von R., Frau Emmy von N., Miss Lucy R.—how, in retrospect, I love their wandering wombs, their tremors and anesthesias. From my days with Charcot to the present, they have done so much for my theory and for sensitizing my cuisine.

Breuer, however, though he joined me in writing our *Studies on Hysteria,* never could truly accept what was so apparent to me, that under the guise of sexuality, food disorder was the great component of all hysterias. Anna O.

would eat only oranges; Dora was "a poor eater and confessed to some disinclination for food"; Miss Lucy R. suffered strange sensations of smell. So, too, that very early case (1893) of the young mother who could not nurse her baby or keep her own food down until I treated her with these hypnotic suggestions: "Do not be afraid. Your stomach is perfectly quiet, your appetite is excellent, you are looking forward to your next meal." The next step in the treatment was to suggest, "she would break out against her family with some acrimony: what had happened to her dinner? did they mean to let her starve? how could she feed the baby if she had nothing to feed herself? and so on."

There was Frau Cecilie M., who suffered from bad teeth and Fräulein Rosalia H., aged twenty-three, who kept feeling a choking sensation in her throat; Fräulein Elisabeth von R.'s trigeminal neuralgia, which was made worse by opening her mouth and chewing—but not talking; Fräulein Katerina, whose throat would close on her when she remembered seeing her uncle lying down with the cook.

And Frau Emmy von N., who had gastric pains that I had to stroke and hypnotize away. Little wonder, since her husband dropped dead one morning at breakfast. One day I called on her at lunchtime while she was surreptitiously throwing something away. She admitted it was her pudding and that she did this every day at lunch. I soon saw that she left most of her food on her plate, justifying this action by saying it was bad for her to eat more, and that her father too was a small eater. She could only drink thick fluids like milk and cocoa; water ruined her digestion. I could go on and on because she and I spent a great deal of time arguing over her dietary habits. Once, after putting her under hypnosis, I finally asked her why she could not eat. She said that when as a child she refused food, she had been punished and forced to eat the meat congealed in its fat, cold, two hours later. "I can still see the fork in front of me . . . one of its prongs was a little bent. Whenever I sit down to a meal I see the plates before me with the cold meat and fat on them."

Anna O. herself was actually a very hungry girl, and Breuer, under the spell of his countertransference and his need to get away for a little Venetian scampi, thought Anna was hungry for him.

This confusion of hungers led to his subsequent prudery in regard to food, and it showed in his cooking. I could not stand the beef dish he and his wife prepared for me on visits to their home. Knowing how I loved beef, and especially when Charcot-broiled, they would nonetheless put only the tiniest pieces on a skewer, interspersed with veritable petticoats of mushrooms, chunks of tomato, and great girdles of onions and peppers, the vegetables completely hiding the meat from the naked eye. It was ridiculous! Brushed with oil, seasoned with fresh marjoram, and carefully roasted, Breuered Beef was quite tasty, but really, one might as well have been a vegetarian. I reasoned with them constantly to expose the beef, or at least cut it bigger on the skewer, but to no avail.

Breuered Beef was enough to make me want to emigrate. I often thought of places where they might have spicier and more interesting sauces for beef, and bigger cuts as well. Unfortunately, they were all in America: Texas with its barbecues, New York with its strip sirloins, and even, I confess, Kansas City with its quarter-pounders. I could not see myself in Kansas City, but it was a thought.

NOTES

Dora "was a poor eater . . ."; *Coll. Papers,* trans. Alix and James Strachey (London: Hogarth, 1925), vol. III, p. 38.
"Do not be afraid . . ."; *Coll. Papers,* vol. V (1950), pp. 36–37.
"Frau Cecilie M"; *Studies on Hysteria, Standard Edition* (London: Hogarth), vol. II, p. 176.
"Fräulein Rosalia H."; ibid., p. 169.
"Fräulein Elisabeth von R."; ibid., p. 178.
"Fräulein Katerina"; ibid., p. 126.
"Frau Emmy von N."; ibid., p. 54, p. 60, pp. 80–82.

BANANA O.

The real name of Anna O. was Bertha Pappenheim, a name lacking *en grande tenue* I thought, except perhaps for an elephant. A catchy *nom de couche* was of course imperative for a famous analyst's patients (just as, if my own name were not Freud—"Joy"—I would have changed it to that). *Nomen est omen.* The public would surely never have taken to heart a case named Bertha Pappenheim any more than it would the case of a Sergius Pankejeff. But "Anna O.," and "The Wolfman," they were winners!

Anna O. suffered all kinds of hysterical symptoms, including the inability to eat anything but oranges. She also had two personalities, one normal and one, as Jones would say, "naughty." Breuer, whose patient she was, went to her house and found that merely by having her describe her symptoms to him, she was relieved of them.

—I can't eat, she told him.

—Oh? he asked, patiently. How long have you felt this way?

—Gee, I'm hungry, she suddenly replied, and started craving a banana that she saw in his lunch pail.

At first Breuer could not decide whether this was a manifestation of the naughty Anna personality. (I have described elsewhere her hysterical pregnancy, with Breuer as the hysterical father: see "Breuered Beef.")

But *vivere est cogitare* and Breuer had an idea.

—Come with me to the kitchen, Anna O., and bring that banana. I think I know a way to prepare it that will not only satisfy your nonexistent appetite, but forever cure you of those other female gripes too.

(Breuer, it must be said, had a way with women. When Martha used to tease me that women patients were falling in love with *me,* I insisted to the contrary: "For that to happen one has to be a Breuer.")

In the kitchen, he bade Anna O. peel the banana, then slice it lengthwise. She sautéed the two halves in a skillet with 2 tbs. melted butter, then added 2 tbs. banana liqueur and 2 tbs. rum. After a minute or two, she removed the banana slices, put them in dishes with scoops of vanilla ice cream, poured the sauce over the top, and served one dish to Breuer and one to herself.

As she swallowed spoonful after spoonful, one could see in her face, Breuer said, the happiness and contentment with life that had hitherto been denied her as a woman.

Thanks to Anna O., the psychotherapeutic armamentarium was enriched with a new method, the talking cure. But as my followers failed to grasp, the talk that cured occurred in the kitchen. Moreover, Anna's banana was neither sublimated into mere talk nor reduced to its symbolic significance, Dr. Breuer's phallus. Sometimes a banana is just a banana.

We could not, however, just call the new culinary creation "Anna's Banana." So, musing well past midnight (and after rising at 6 A.M., breakfast at 7, 1st patient at 8, my walk at 12, lunch at 1, 9th patient at 6 P.M., dinner at 7, cards with Minna at 8, and letter writing since 10), I finally pronounced this little *délice,* "Banana O." And it has made all the difference.

NOTES

". . . as Jones would say, 'naughty' "; Jones, *Life and Work,* vol. 1, p. 224.
"For that to happen . . ."; Jones, ibid., p. 225.

MEMORY SCREEN

We often forget what ingredients, derived from day residues or leftovers, have gone into a soup, especially if the concoction has first been processed in a blender. One needs to sift or screen out unwanted remnants that may remind one of meals past. Hence every kitchen should have this invaluable piece of equipment. It is also good for purees, where one needs a Memory Screen to catch the bitter lemon seeds, the parsley stalks, and the peppercorns.

SPLIT FLIESS SOUP

If you find yourself stirring this soup with your left hand, beware! Fliess, my dear invaluable writing companion during that most important decade in my life, the 1890s, had a theory of the universal bisexuality of the human race, where left-handed people figured most perversely. Furthermore, he had a bizarre theory of "periodic laws," in which the numbers 28 and 23 kept recurring. The number 28, based on the period of menstruation, was the feminine component, and the number 23, based on the interval between the close of one menstrual period and the beginning of the next, was the masculine one. For Fliess, these numbers determined everything: birth, death, gender, the rhythms of life, when one would develop appendicitis, when one would burn the bacon, etc. I could not accept such nonpsychological determinism, of course, but I made his theory of bisexuality, nonetheless, an important cornerstone in my psychoanalytic theory, and Split Fliess Soup an important element in my cuisine.

It was because of this theory, however, that our friendship terminated, I regret to say, most bitterly. Fliess claimed that a patient of mine plagiarized the Fliess bisexuality theory before he could himself publish it, and that the "leak," as he called it, came through me. I admitted as much, but it was because of this that Fliess never wrote to me again. What would he say, were he alive today, if he learned that I was herewith giving away his soup recipe too!

Soak the peas in batches of 23 or 28 at a time (their hulls removed, they cook more quickly than whole peas) for several hours in cold water. Simmer them in 3 cups water, stirring until they virtually dissolve. While simmering, Fliess would add, in what he thought was sexual symmetry, a chopped seeded tomato and a leftover ham bone. Remove the ham bone and puree the soup in a food processor. Return to stove and add a little cream or stock to thicken. Season with salt and pepper and serve.

Fliess would only make this between the 23rd and 28th of the month, but I have found such idiosyncratic precautions unnecessary.

KRAEPELIN SUZETTES

Why did everyone always defer to Kraepelin? Jones went off to study with him; Jung could not stop arguing with him; and even my dear Wolfman saw him in Munich for therapy. Kraepelin, Zeppelin! So he was the most organized thinker in psychiatry and author of its classic textbook. I still outlived him, though we were born in the same year. Besides, his term *dementia praecox* did not last; the Swiss took care of that by replacing it with schizophrenia, a typically Zurich term for a typically Zurich syndrome! As for Kraepelin, he is today mere history. The only thing an ordinary psychiatrist still uses from his textbook is this recipe, which was the reward of his scientific conscientiousness. As Janet had his Madeleine, Jung his crazy Babette, so Kraepelin had his Suzette, on whose case he did a long-term follow-up study, tracing her to her kitchen, thirty years later, where he found her, pan in hand, still smiling dementedly as in her youth. She immediately served him these pancakes, and he smiled too.

> In a chafing dish, melt $^1/_2$ cup butter with 4 tsp. sugar. Add the juice of an orange and 3 tbs. of Grand Marnier. Boil to bubbling. Put 2 or 3 crêpes (per person) in sauce and turn, folding crêpes. Pour a tbs. of cognac over each, and when just precocious enough to ignite, ignite and serve.

THE INTERPRETATION OF CREAMS

The most valuable of all discoveries it has been my good fortune to make was the Interpretation of Creams. Insight such as this falls to one's lot but once in a lifetime. The prescientific conception of creams which obtains among the French, for example, is in perfect keeping with their perverse conception of the universe.

The French take a half pint of fresh cream and ferment it by adding a tablespoon of either sour cream or yogurt, leaving this mixture (in a covered dish) to mature for a day before chilling. The final product, cultured and ripened, is called by the French *crème fraîche*, which means, perversely, "fresh cream."

Then there is the peculiar dish called *crème anglaise*. It is really nothing but a custard sauce, made by sadistically beating four egg yolks with a half cup sugar and a painful pinch of cornstarch until thickened. A pint of hot milk is slowly stirred in, then the whole mixture placed on the stove over moderate heat and stirred until thick. Where is the cream? There isn't any!

This accounts for the main impression made by "creams" after one has eaten them: the manifest cream so disguises its latent content that the cream seems to be something alien, coming, as it were, from another world, or at least from another country.

Take Bavarian cream, for example. It has nothing to do with Bavaria, land of *Biergartens* and *Weisswurst,* and that is my point. It is really the aforementioned *crème anglaise,* to which is added a half ounce gelatin mixed with a little orange juice (or chocolate or strawberry sauce or whatever sweet flavoring you desire). Five beaten egg whites are stirred in, the mixture chilled, and then a quarter pint of viciously whipped cream added later. Hardly Bavarian, except for the latent violence, yet this little *Schatz* of a dessert, usually turned out in a ring mold and chilled again before serving, is delicious.

It is interesting to note that in Bavaria they have replied to this very English dessert by adapting it to Germanic tastes and naming the result, perversely again, "Norfolk cream." For Norfolk cream, a mold is lined with candied fruits, especially plums. Bavarian cream, mixed with some candied cherries, is then poured into the mold and, when served, garnished with whipped cream.

The Americans, at least when I visited the Stanley Halls in Worcester, Massachusetts, also do astonishing things with creams, though they are not, at least so far, as nationalistic about them as we Europeans. Perhaps they are not yet discontent enough with their civilization.

Americans divide cream into light, medium, heavy, and sour, as well as some borderline phenomenon I have never quite understood called "half-and-half," a compromise formation which masks both cream and milk. Also available is a whipping cream which is not, as one might first expect, the same as their heavy cream. If this seems confusing, it is further complicated by the fact that American light cream is far to be preferred in cooking European recipes that call for cream, though many Americans seem to think heavy cream is intended in these, perhaps because of their association of all things European with "heavy."

G. Stanley Hall made us a delightful Newport cream (named for the summer resort in Rhode Island). He whipped together a pint of sour cream, a half cup of milk, the juice of half a lemon, and a little rum.

Newport cream at least had the authenticity of being from Newport. It would be an error to suppose, however, that the old theory of the alien origin of creams lacks followers even in our own times. Mystical cooks (Maurice-Edmond Sailland, for example, whose slavophilia led him to change his name to Curnonsky, the first two syllables being the Latin for "Why not?" and the last syllable an attempt to bring him closer to his beloved Russian creams) cling, as they are perfectly justified in doing, to the remnants of the once-predominant nationalistic interpretation of creams. These jingoistic "remnants," however, must soon be swept away by scientific explanation. And we not infrequently find that quite intelligent persons, who in other respects are averse to anything of a romantic nature (Brillat-Savarin, for example, who wrote many volumes on politics and law in addition to his famed compendium on the art of dining), still go so far as to base their culinary belief in the existence of divine powers in the phenomena of creams. Some of these otherwise rational writers even continue to believe in the divinity of creams which prevailed in antiquity, talking of "divine" or "inspired" creams.

But as I have not succeeded in mastering the whole of this literature—indeed I would hardly have had time for my patients or other writing if I attempted to review all the literature on creams—I must ask my readers to rest content with the story of my original breakthrough in cream interpretation.

It was in the Schloss Belle Vue, a restaurant, on 24 July 1895, that I first glimpsed, through the analysis of a dessert that had just been served me, my future theory that the essence of a cream is the fulfillment of a hidden wish.

Dessert that warm afternoon was called Charlotte Malakoff, a quite suggestive concoction in which delicate sponge fingers, dipped in liqueur, line the sides of a mold. An almond cream, consisting of a little butter and sugar, a spritz of almond extract, some chopped almonds, and a shot of liqueur, all beaten together with a pint of whipped cream, are poured over the mold in layers with more and more sponge fingers, then chilled.

As I sat there, in the Belle Vue, contemplating the case of Charlotte M., I noticed that it was served with still another whipped cream on top, called *crème Chantilly*. What ruse was going on, I pondered, with this Charlotte Russe? Why Chantilly? I asked myself. What does this fragrant Russian woman have to do with a little village in France famous for lace? Or is lace the connection? In that case, should not the *crème Chantilly* be served under the Charlotte M., instead of on top? Did she wear her lace on her head, this alcoholic Russian aristocrat?

But what is *crème Chantilly?* I asked myself. Surely it is nothing more than soundly whipped cream, with a spoonful of sugar and vanilla extract added. It is what in Vienna, in our more honest moments at least, we simply call *Schlag* (though without sugar or vanilla), meaning beater, or beating instrument. Ah hah! I said. Charlotte Malakoff indeed! These geographical cream names are nothing but disguises, repressions for something so deeply obscene, and yet so clearly wished for, namely, sumptuously pampered taste buds, that the culinary imagination must project them out of one's own country and onto another.

Thus the French, who invented *crème anglaise*, name

it for the English. The English blame Bavarians or Russians for their creams. Germans respond to the English with great salvos of creams, usually attacking by way of France. Only in Vienna, I am proud to say, have we had the honesty to call a *Schlag* a *Schlag*. We have always kept the whip in whipped cream. (Unlike, I might add, the French, who name this phenomenon for one of their obscure noblemen, as if sadism were somehow their invention and property! "Sadism" is a chauvinism—whipping originated in Vienna, also the home of Sacher-Masoch, and like masochism, should rightly be named oberism, from *Schlag Obers,* which is Viennese for whipped cream *on top.*)

How much of this streak in Austrian creams is due to the Spanish Hapsburg influence, I cannot speculate. One dish left by the Hapsburg dynasty, however, that still appears occasionally even in the best Viennese families, is called *crème dementia.* The work, no doubt, of some Velázquez dwarf, it calls for the dissolving of a package of gelatin in a cup of boiling water; meanwhile, a custard of three beaten egg yolks mixed with a tablespoon sugar and a dwarf pinch of salt is thickened in the top of a Double-Bleuler with a cup of hot milk. The gelatin water is added, along with three severely beaten egg whites and a teaspoon sherry. The mixture is chilled in serving dishes, and each finally topped with a teaspoon of crème de menthe.

On this question, then, of whether creams should be acquitted of evil, there is no end of discussion. No longer, however, would I expose creams to reductive analysis. If *"Traum,"* as we say in German, *"ist nur Schaum,"* cream, too, is only foam.

I cannot, in other words, agree with the poet Yeats that "in creams begin responsibilities." Creams may be immoral, sinful even, the manifest cream merely a disguise for hidden contents, but nothing that is ethically offensive in our creamlife need truly trouble us. No one should experience the least sense of guilt over creams. As with so much else in our psyches, creams are *köstlich,* delicious, a joy to be savored by all. We are such stuff as creams are made of, and our little bodies rounded by desserts.

WISH-FULFILLMENT ICING

In a saucepan combine all the sugar you want (1 cup will do a cake), about the same amount of water, 1 tbs. corn syrup, and a dash of salt. Boil, stirring gently, until it thickens. Cool. In top of your Double-Bleuler, melt all the chocolate you want (5 oz. will do a cake) with 1 tsp. strong coffee per oz. of chocolate. Stir in about the same amount of butter as chocolate. Pour out a glass of rum and add half to the chocolate. Sip the other half while stirring chocolate mixture into cooled syrup. When cool, blend in 1/3 cup whipped cream. Stir until both icing and you feel smooth.

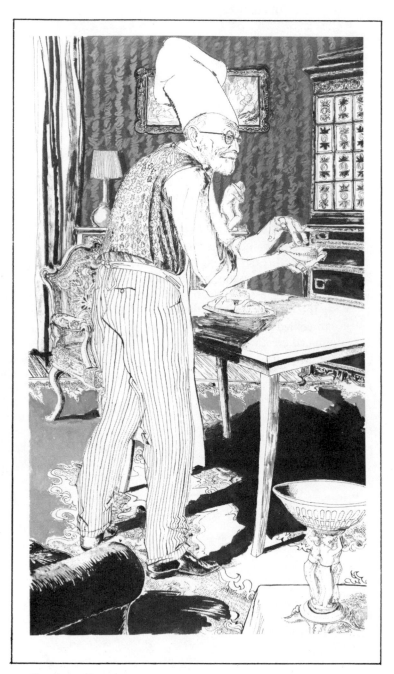

Erogenous Scones

V.

MY FAVORITES

Erogenous Scones, Incredible Oedipal Pie, Little Hansburgers, and the Like

"Minna is resting in her room, I am thinking of eating a pomegranate. . . ."
—Letter to the family, 25 September 1908, in *Letters of Sigmund Freud, 1873–1939*, ed. E. L. Freud

EROGENOUS SCONES

Not until my 1905 work, *Three Essays on the Theory of Sexuality,* were the erogenous zones of the human body removed from the secrecy of the bedroom to the public arena of science. Each zone yields its specific excitation and, eventually, character style: the oral with its desire for immediate gratification, which gives the base for all the sucking, licking, and biting pleasures; the anal, with its pleasure in tension and retention and which gives the base for delayed, obsessional, and controlled pleasures. In hysterical persons, these body zones and neighboring tracts and mucous membranes take on the excitations of the actual genitalia, so that eating, swallowing, digesting, and excreting can become orgasmic. Almost any area of the body can become an erogenous zone (in sadomasochism it is the skin; in voyeurism and exhibitionism it is the eye).

I wish the same could be said for scones, but the way most people make them drives one to despair. They always seem to lack the erogenous touch. Look around the kitchen for berries, ground clove, cherries, skins of lemons or oranges, cinnamon, etc.

> Make a basic unerogenous scone dough by mixing 3 cups flour, 2 tbs. sugar, 1 tsp. baking powder, 1/2 tsp. baking soda, 1 stick butter, and 1 cup of milk. Now add an erogenous touch (for some this need only be a cherry, macerated into the dough). Roll out the dough to a thickness of 1/2 inch and cut out the scones into erotic shapes (for some, a leg, for others a nice heart-shaped derrière—you must use your imagination or it will not be erogenous). Bake on greased baking sheet in 400° oven for about 15 minutes.

INCREDIBLE OEDIPAL PIE

I had no true realization, when first recording this rather modest recipe, how long it would last or what a cliché it was destined to become in every kitchen. The pie is edible, but its fame incredible. Nowadays, people just call it "Mom's Apple Pie." In October 1897, while digging ever deeper into the sources of my own neuroses, and writing off theories to my friend Wilhelm Fliess in Berlin (Fliess, by the way, had a superb nose for interesting combinations, being a famous nose-and-throat man himself—see Split Fliess Soup), I remembered my childhood despair, "crying my heart out, because my mother was nowhere to be found."

Soon I found "love of the mother and jealousy of the father to be a general phenomenon of early childhood." How simple the formula! Yet it would be a long time before I would recognize the simplicity of Oedipal Pie. No one can resist this dish because, as I said to Fliess, as children we were each "once a budding Oedipus in phantasy."

Mix 1 cup sugar, 2 tbs. flour, dash of salt, several sliced apples (peeled and cored), 1/2 cup raisins, 1/2 cup chopped walnuts, 3 tbs. dark rum, and a half stick of butter melted. Meanwhile, and best of all if she is standing by watching you make this, ask your mother for her favorite pie crust recipe, and line a pie pan with this crust. Add apple mixture, and cover with crust. Bake in 450° oven for 10 minutes, then reduce temperature to 350° and bake 25 minutes more. Cool to room temperature. And don't forget your mother.

NOTES
"crying my heart out"; "love of the mother"; "once a budding Oedipus"; letter to Fliess, 15 October 1897.

LITTLE HANSBURGERS

The case of Little Hans, with its story of a child's sexual fantasies, remains to this day an unshakable cornerstone of our new science—but what turmoil, what outrage, what anger it caused! Contrary to current opinion, however, this hue and cry was not due to some imagined violation of the sexual strictures of Victorian society. Furthermore, the horde of five-year-olds who suddenly started giving testimony, most of it silly, to all sorts of sophisticated erotic experiences was not the result, as many think, of unconscious suggestion on the part of their adult interrogators.

And when I wrote that "I never got a finer insight into a child's soul," I did not mean by this what so many have concluded, that my theories of infantile sexuality were thereby confirmed. Here is what really happened.

Little Hans, the precocious four-and-a-half-year-old son of one of my disciples, was already preoccupied with people or animals that had "widdlers," as he called the phallic organ. When he saw a horse drop in its tracks in the street, he developed a phobia of being bitten by a horse. But the cure came easily, once we penetrated to his precocious insight into a first law of nature: dead horses, like all dead animals, are meat. The cure required a symbolic enactment of another law of nature: eat or be eaten. (One law of nature cures another law of nature: *Similia similibus curantur.*)

I told his mother, to whom of course Widdle Hans (as I liked to call him) was singularly attached, to prepare for him a medium-rare hamburger made of horsemeat, and to encourage him to bite into it savagely. His father, meanwhile, took notes of everything he did and said.

When I saw the boy years later, he remembered nothing of his childhood, neither horses, nor fears, nor his father's note-taking. But all he wanted to eat was Hansburgers! Hansburgers and more Hansburgers! And suddenly every child in Austria, every child in Europe, wanted Hansburgers and nothing else. They started making up all kinds of erotic fantasies in the hope of receiving the same treatment Widdle Hans got.

That was the source of the outrage against my theories—not by a Victorian society whose smugness was threatened by the theory of infantile sexuality—but by parents of good taste and varied diet who saw in me, correctly I now confess, the source of their children's maniacal craving for that bestial food. The father of psychoanalysis? *Nein!* I am the father of the Hansburger.

If you like horsemeat, as we Europeans do, use it. Otherwise, you may use ordinary ground beef, but you will not know what you are missing. Shape meat into little phallic loaves like sausages and cook to medium rare. Serve each on a widdle bun.

NOTES

"I never got a finer insight . . ."; Jones, *Life and Work,* vol. 2, p. 294.

WIT PILAFFS

One day I was visited by a young Viennese woman, Frau H., wife of a rice merchant of my acquaintance, who complained of an embarrassing disturbance in her laugh-life. Frequently, and ever-increasingly, when she broke into laughter, she would wet her pants. Sitting in her salon at home, or gaily bantering with friends at a café, flirting and joking, she would suddenly rise up and race off, only to arrive at her intended goal too late to avert the inevitable catastrophe. (It was the case of Frau H., in fact, that led me for the first time in my practice to place the patient on a couch, in a supine position, thereby hoping to relieve pressure on the bladder and save my carpets.)

The reader will readily assume that the symptom has its origins in childhood bed-wetting during sleep. But this path toward understanding defies the logic of the unconscious. For uproarious laughter does not usually accompany wetting one's bed, even in sleep, and only the most infantile *Schlemozzle* would find laughter in wetting the bed in childhood.

The symptom encroached evermore upon my patient's intimate life. Formerly gay and carefree, with happy eyes, she came to my consulting room grimly wrapped in a strange garment, which she believed could be opened the more quickly in an emergency. Every nerve in her face defended against even the slightest potential for humor.

She could no longer attend the comic opera, she said, missing as well the sardonic comedies of our famous Wiener, Schnitzler. In fact, she refused all theater save for Racine. Her husband was condemned to telling her only lugubrious tales of business dealings, and recently she had taken to wearing padding in her underclothes. Her laughlife was seriously disturbed.

I must here break into the narrative to inform the reader that her symptom, though I had then not yet met it in my practice, was epidemic in Vienna during the so-called "Belle Epoque." The bustling life of the coffee houses, the hurriedness of the music halls and the fast pace of the *Weingartens* was not just due to the legendary Viennese wit and merriment. For accompanying this wit and merriment was an incontinent urge to pee that went with one's laugh. A ceaseless flow in and around the tables was of laughing ladies hastening to and from their *Toiletten*.

Here, then, was a symptom that threw together two involuntary reactions of the nervous system. What on the

— 79 —

level of the psyche, I asked myself, corresponded with these involuntary nervous reactions? What, in other words, was the unconscious association of peeing and laughing?

The "pilaff," as I later termed this syndrome, provided the impetus for my long study on humor, *Wit and Its Relation to the Unconscious,* in 1905. There I was able to record for my own amusement, under the guise of a "scientific" analysis, of course, my favorite anecdotes and stories, which were to keep me laughing into late old age.

Crucial to all such cases is what I wrote there: "Strictly speaking, we do not know what we are laughing about."

We do know, however, that repression is the soul of wit, and that sudden laughter represents the breakthrough of the deeply repressed. The common denominator of the pilaff, then, is a holding back of the repressed. Amelioration of the symptom is thus only possible, as I learned from this case, by lifting the repression in stages and by gradually easing into the joke.

Frau H. had hitherto always "burst" into laughter, or she would "break" into laughter or be overcome by spasms of it. She had fallen prey to the quick wit of one-liners, or "quickies" as she called them. She had to learn through analysis to move slowly from wit to humor.

Unlike wit, humor extends over an entire situation satisfying one deeply; it is not concentrated at a single point of explosive discharge. Her defense against all humor had only increased its tendency to appear the more urgently. She learned in analysis to sublimate her holding back into delay, a sublimation that allowed ripples of pleasure and small bubbles of joy to precede the climactic punch line which could be delayed interminably as she simmered her laughter slowly.

I termed this "the forepleasure principle." This refers to laughter in anticipation of joking, laughter that there is a joke going on, or laughter for its own sake. This case taught me that the content of the repression is nothing other than the laugh itself, a fact I have ever and again confirmed. No, it is not the genital aspect of the laughable that is repressed but the laughable aspect of the genitals. What is repressed is laughter itself and what cures must therefore also be the return of the repressed, the repressed laugh.

One is reduced to laughter, I see now, and not the other way around. The error of my wit book was in my attempt to reduce laughter to something else: sexual libido. Laughter is the irreducible, all human: all people have it. There are even taboos on it; but that is another subject.

The charming young woman, having refound her "irrepressible" joy in life, discovered in analysis the art of the forepleasure principle, drawing out the jokes into ever more witty refinements, and seeing in advance what was coming down the *Strasse,* so to speak. Now she could imagine the endings and not need to arrive there so quickly, enjoying instead minor flourishes and delicious titillations along the way.

Years later I learned that she left the rice merchant and Vienna, too, and had a noteworthy career in American vaudeville on the Steel Pier in Atlantic City.

The following pilaff recipes, then, all the product of this patient's analysis, with occasional pleasurable trips to the kitchen to work them out, will be tried by the patient cook. Remember, in your patience is your soul. There are no rice shortcuts, I have found. A diet of minute rice is as cloying as having to listen to a string of one-liners. One may laugh, but not well. Let the pilaff cook. Let the pun rise.

NOTE
"Strictly speaking . . ."; *Wit and Its Relation to the Unconscious,* trans. A. A. Brill in *The Basic Writings of Sigmund Freud* (New York: Random House, 1938), p. 697.

WIT PILAFF # 1 (WITH CHICKEN LIVERS)

Chop a couple of onions until you start crying and
someone comes in and asks you why you are crying.
Say something dramatic, like, you just can't take it
anymore, life is too hard and miserable, or that you
cannot live without love. Proceed to sauté the onions
in butter, along with a few tbs. of finely chopped
carrot and celery. After several minutes toss in a few
good squirmy handfuls of duly chopped chicken livers,
and another handful of mushrooms, browning them
for about 5 minutes. Stir in 2 cups raw rice and ½
cup of sherry and cook until absorbed. (Drink the
other ½ cup while you're waiting—remember: Wit
Pilaffs are fun or they are nothing!) Add 2 cups of
chicken broth, salt, pepper, bay leaf, and a pinch of
thyme, oregano, or your favorite herb. Cook over low
heat until all liquid is absorbed and serve topped with
grated Parmesan.

WIT PILAFF # 2 (WITH SHRIMP)

This recipe is fun if you are the father of a boy who is
having an Oedipal crisis. The night before you make
it, announce to the family that you need a little
shrimp for a Wit Pilaff that you are going to make.
This will give the youngster something to think
about. Next day, heat a few tbs. of olive oil with a few
tbs. of butter and sauté, briefly, a minced clove of
garlic with 1 cup raw rice. Add ½ cup vermouth and
cook until absorbed. Add 2 cups chicken broth and
cook for several minutes, covered. Meanwhile, call out
to your son, "Come here, you little shrimp!" and
when he does, just smile and give him a good old-
fashioned knuckle-rub on the top of his little head. He
will be so relieved, he will laugh. Then have him shell
and devein a pound of uncooked shrimp (counsel him

that it will be good experience). When the rice has
about 5 minutes to go, add the shrimp along with salt,
pepper, and a smack of marjoram. Recover and cook
for another 10 minutes, or until all the broth is
absorbed and your son is recovered too.

THE DOUBLE-BLEULER

The origins of this instrument are said to go back to the
bain-marie, or Mary's bath, of early alchemy, where it was
used to provide a prolonged gentle heat for dissolving immersed substances. "Mary" was the legendary Maria
Prophetessa of Egypt, another name for Miriam, the sister
of Moses. Because the alchemists also referred to Maria as
Mary the Jewess, the history of refined cooking indeed
commences in the art of the Jewish mother.

But the Double-Bleuler we use is a Swiss piece of
equipment: a smaller, thinner pot sits concealed inside a
sturdier one of solid reputation, whose bottom is well-cov-
ered, so as to prevent the contents inside from direct con-
tact with the heat. Martha uses it for melting chocolate
that might otherwise burn or for sauces that tend to curdle
or separate.

The Double-Bleuler takes its name from old Eugen
Bleuler's famous theory of ambivalence. He coined the
term in 1910 for those double tendencies of the will and
emotion in schizophrenia, when, as he said, the "patients
want at the same time to eat and not to eat."

Others more privy to Bleuler, the man, maintain that
the concept of two pots under one lid refers to his own
character. He was a very concealing man, so thick-skinned
and stiff that, as I said once, "it's like embracing a piece of
linoleum."

But I know those Swiss! The Double-Bleuler is just

clever Swiss shorthand for Eugen and his little son Manfred, who grew up in the Burghölzli Clinic among his father's patients. The *klein* Bleuler also became a psychiatrist, but was not as big as his father. Always, with Swiss equipment, one has to be careful: they like to give things a mystique sometimes that is neither necessary nor deserved.

NOTES

"it's like embracing . . ."; *The Freud/Jung Letters,* ed. William McGuire, trans. Ralph Manheim and R. F. C. Hull (Princeton: Bollingen, 1974), F/253.

". . . to eat and not to eat."; Eugen Bleuler, *A Textbook of Psychiatry,* trans. A. A. Brill (New York: Dover, 1924, 1951), p. 382.

WORD SALAD
(*Wortsalat*)

So much craziness has come into our field from only one or two places. The Burghölzli, that crazy-house in Zurich, was a nut factory of untold influence on the future of psychopathology. Eugen Bleuler was in charge there, and Jung was one of his assistants.

Bleuler observed that schizophrenics—the bread and butter of the Burghölzli's business—spoke dissociated words that none of his staff could understand. A "word salad," he called it in his textbook. Jung tried to help out by stringing words together with his association experiments. But they were both wrong: Word Salad does not refer to words, it refers to salad.

Bleuler obviously invented the term by analogy with the cut-up lettuce that is doused in sour, salty dressing and served by the Swiss as a side dish in institutional meals. (I know, because when I visited Jung there, he put me up, not at the Baur-au-lac but at the Burghölzli itself.)

Bleuler, who did not even drink beer, would have found even the conversation at an office party incomprehensible. How could he expect to understand schizophrenic talk when he did not even understand how to make an interesting salad? Oh, those Swiss, what I have had to put up with from them!

How many times must I say it: patients are not off their noodles, it is their noodles that are off. A good Word Salad shows this.

> Place a package of noodles in a pot of boiling water (do not use those crazy twisted pasta shells: they are only for psychotic Italian salads and will not work in our northern European ones). Cook only until tender. Place the drained noodles in a salad bowl which you have previously rubbed with garlic cloves. Add a few slices of tomatoes, sweet peppers, scallions, a small can of tuna—or use other seafood or shellfish if your institution can afford them (and even the poorest budget can sneak in an anchovy now and then)— some olives, a handful of chopped basil or at least parsley, and salt and pepper. Dress the salad with olive oil and gently stir. Refrigerate until shortly before serving and then top with a few chopped nuts (if you have to ask what kind, perhaps you should not be making a *Wortsalat:* stick with plain lettuce).

NOTE
"in his textbook"; Bleuler, *A Textbook of Psychiatry,* pp. 155, 398.

FETTUCCINE LIBIDO

Libido, as I pointed out in my *Three Essays on the Theory of Sexuality* (1905), is fundamentally masculine in nature.

Consequently, sexuality in men is a rather simple, perhaps an all too simple, matter. It is more complex, perhaps too complex, in women, which explains women's greater predisposition to hysteria, a matter I am loath to bring up in the present hysterical climate on this subject, except to say that when it comes to fettuccine, especially in this recipe, women should probably not try to make it. Nor, for that matter, should men.

Since Fliess long ago convinced me of the fundamental bisexuality of human beings, I think the ideal chef for Fettuccine Libido is a homosexual. Only homosexuals seem to have the right combination of simple masculine libido with complex feminine libido. I have found this true over and over again at the superior restaurants of the world, where homosexuals always seem to be the chefs or the waiters, or both.

If only I had realized this when I was writing my now-famous letter to the despairing mother of a homosexual in America, I would have told that lady to quit complaining and be thankful her son could make her a Fettuccine Libido! Homosexuals seem to have a predilection for it. They make it so much it borders on Fettuccism. But that is all right with me. I cannot get enough of it either.

> Cook the fettuccine for about 10 minutes, or until it is
> *al dente.* While it is cooking, melt a stick of unsalted
> butter in a saucepan, stirring in until smooth 1/4 cup
> flour and 1/4 cup grated Parmesan cheese. Slowly add
> 1 cup hot cream and continue stirring. In a separate
> pan, saute 1/2 cup cooked peas with a few slices of
> diced prosciutto. Add to the sauce. Drain the
> fettuccine and toss with the sauce. Serve with a
> flourish, if you can find one.

NOTE
"my now famous letter"; see Jones, *Life and Work,* vol. 3, pp. 195–196.

THE RATMAN'S CHEESECAKE

This recipe dates from October 1907. A young man, with university education no less, came to my consulting room to resolve severe obsessions, including slashing his own throat with a razor, and, most vividly and alarmingly, his obsession with the idea that a rat was boring its way into the anus of his father, and of an admired woman. Treatment followed the association method. I made the patient say everything that came into his mind, even if unpleasant to him, or seemingly unimportant or irrelevant. Nonetheless, nothing could have surprised me more than what came out. It was the following delicious recipe, which I, seated out of his sight, immediately copied down.

A package of crushed chocolate wafers, of course, are *de rigueur* for the crust, although we used zwieback crumbs too. Mix with 1/2 cup of melted butter and 2 tbs. sugar. Press crumbs to cover bottom of cake pan. Melt 12 oz. bittersweet chocolate with half a stick of butter. Cool. Beat into 1 1/2 lbs. of cream cheese; gradually add 2 tbs. rum, 3 egg yolks, 1/2 cup sugar and a razor's edge of salt. Pour into crust. Bake in 325° oven for an hour, or until center is set when tested with a knife. (Watch that knife!) Top with chopped nuts and serve chilled.

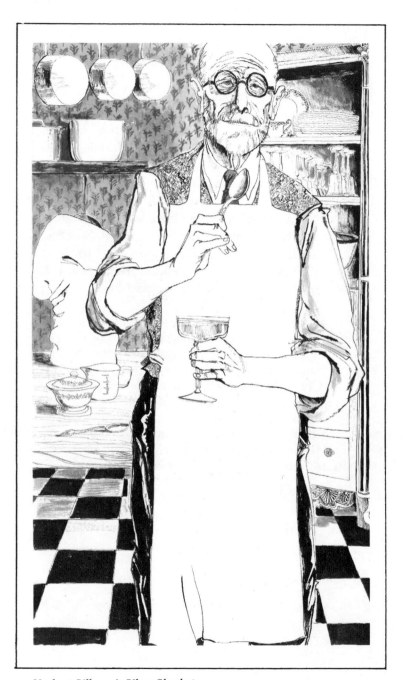

Herbert Silberer's Silver Sherbet

VI.

WEDNESDAY EVENING SNACKS

From Sublimation Sandwiches (Subs) to Frau Lou's Salomé Platter

"News in brief: the coffee here is delicious. . . ."
—Letter to Martha, 19 December 1885,
in *Letters of Sigmund Freud,*
1873–1939, ed. E. L. Freud

Rumors, legends, superstitions—but no scientific evidence can confirm that the "sub" developed from the Hoagie which in turn developed from "Hog Island" in the Delaware River near Philadelphia in the American Commonwealth of Pennsylvania, where Italian immigrants, who worked in the shipyards there, piled into a loaf of Italian bread slices of cheese, cold cuts, and onions together with salads, pickles, and peppers, and the omnipotent tomato (see also "The Birth of the Myth of the Hero").

The Americans unscrupulously claim priority in field after field, even the sandwich, and in this regard their chauvinism and plagiarism can be compared only with that of their most feared rivals, the Russians (a perfect example of repression of one's own character deficiencies and projection of them upon a supposed enemy).

No, the sandwich as a sublimation actually began at our Wednesday meetings of the *Psychoanalytische Vereinigung* when I and my first few loyal disciples met in the evenings to discuss cases and ideas. After all, what time did we have for dinner? None. We came straight from our practices, hungry. In those days we could not just send out for a pizza, and if we could, do you think Adler would have been willing to be a go-fer? or Eitingon? Such neighborhood conveniences were simply not available in our *Bezirk*. We had to sublimate our appetites for home-cooked meals of *Gulaschsuppe* and *Aprikosenknödel,* so we brought with us our personal sandwiches, each a symbolic sublimation of what we might have been satisfied with at home.

As time went on, we brought ever-larger sandwiches and even began to trade among ourselves, for such was the closeness of the original circle (before Adler and Stekel betrayed the filial affection). A bit of roast beef from Stekel for the sliced pickles in Sachs' loaf, or the delicious cold *Leberkäs* of Eitingon against some of my Liptauer cheese which Minna (or was it Martha?) had so thoughtfully packed. It was so hard in those days to keep the *Fettflecken* or mustard off the latest issues of *Imago*.

Once, when this handing around of cold cuts and tasting of one another's delicacies had completely interrupted the discussions of our newest sexual theories, Lou Salomé was so infuriated at our messiness and inattention (and not being one herself to enter the process of sublimation) that she developed her now famous Salomé platter and passed it around (see "Frau Lou's Salomé Platter").

STEKEL TARTARE

"Moral insanity" was how I finally had to characterize Wilhelm Stekel's work. He was conscienceless, making up cases, inventing patients. Every time we brought up a new subject at our Wednesday evening meetings of the Society, Stekel would remark, "Only this morning I saw a case of this kind." We used to call them "Stekel's Wednesday patients."

He wrote a paper once on the psychological significance that people's surnames have in determining their choice of careers, and cited a large number of patients whose names had determined their vocations. When I asked him how he could in conscience publish the names of his patients, he said not to worry, he had made them all up!

In public lectures he used to cite episodes from his life that, from his analysis with me, I knew were untrue, and he would stare at me as if defying me to contradict him and thus break my professional discretion.

He would justify his arrogance by saying of our relationship that a dwarf on the shoulder of a giant sees farther than the giant. "That may be true," I told him, "but a louse on the head of an astronomer does not."

For all I know, he also made up all the fetishes and aberrations he wrote about, all those unsavory stories of silk, satin, and furs, of petticoats and rubber cushions, aprons and ladies' gloves, and leather—oh, the leather! They were all, I think now, Stekel's own fantasies.

He would not admit to making up the recipe for Stekel Tartare, which I have since seen served in many restaurants. He claimed it was acquired by him from a patient whose particular fetish was a roughcast concoction of embryonic meat. But since it was all Stekel ever ate, we can assume this is yet another of his misrepresentations.

> Mix 1 lb. of raw ground steak with an egg, a pinch of salt, a grind of fresh pepper, a smack of G. Stanley Hall's Worcester Sauce, a shoeful of chopped parsley, a few feeling tsp. of dry or prepared mustard, a slap of Tabasco sauce, a finely chopped onion, a mashed clove of garlic, and any other hot seasoning you fancy. Beat the meat gently but firmly in your hands until it is smooth and creamy. Serve as an hors d'oeuvre on toast, but remember, you will not want a main course after it.

NOTES
"Moral insanity . . ."; Jones, *Life and Work,* vol. 2, p. 137.
"Only this morning . . ."; Jones, ibid., p. 135.
"he had made them all up . . . "; Jones, ibid., pp. 135–136.
"but a louse on the head of an astronomer . . ."; Jones, ibid., p. 136.

BRILLED LAMB CHOPS

Abraham Arden Brill, the inventor of this recipe, was an expert in necrophilia. Some years after founding the New York Psycho-Analytic Society, he was in a position to write the definitive psychoanalytical essay on the perverse attraction to dead bodies. He was also the first to translate me into English, and, despite knowing my work so thoroughly, he remained loyal for forty years: from 1908 when he attended our Vienna meetings until his death in 1948. He was one of the few of our group with a genuine culinary background: his father had been a commissary officer in the Imperial Army.

So, even if Jones and Putnam kept telling me that Brill's mangled English was killing my work, and therefore necrophiliac in intention, his translations were faithful to the original, me, and I remained faithful to him. I never threw out our Brill, long after it rusted.

> Before placing on Brill, season lamb chops with salt,
> pepper, lemon juice, and rosemary, making slits in
> the meat to insert the rosemary. But caution! Do not
> overcook and kill the meat. If you use a Double-A
> Brill, get the heat up fast, and keep the chops on no
> more than 2 minutes per quarter inch.

THE BIRTH OF THE MYTH OF THE HERO

This is the best book available on the sandwich. "Little Rank," as I usually referred to him in my letters to others, outdid himself with this one—and I stand fast with that judgment even if he, too, alas, later deserted our community and set up his own diner in New York (*Otto's*). This was the origin of the phrase "rank outsider," which we used to describe forevermore all those who broke with our authority.

No doubt Rank's exhaustive research into the Hero provided adequate compensation to his small stature so that he could finally go off on his own. Actually he was not that much shorter than the others. Jones, too, was a small man, and so were Brill, Ferenczi, and Eitingon. That is why I liked Jung, Hall, and Groddeck so much. They were Hero-sized.

Rank showed that all sandwiches glorify their origins, investing their births with fantastical features. How many silly tales have we heard of the 4th Earl of Sandwich himself, from whom the term supposedly comes. To say nothing of the Hoagie (see "Subs"), the Hot Dog (see "H. W. Frinkfurters"), or the Hansburger. But "sandwich" is a misnomer, a typical appropriation by British chauvinism of the Ur-sandwich, which was a Reuben. Reuben was the first-born son of Jacob by Leah, and from him have come such mythically blessed descendants as ham and cheese (not necessarily Swiss) on rye, with pickle and just a little mustard but no tomato, and the hot pastrami.

Pastrami's legend I find hardly credible. Some contend that he (Giorgiu) was supposed to have been a Rumanian patriot who fled to America to escape Cossack persecution. A pogrom was then raging, trying to force Ukrainian food, what there was of it, onto the Jews, forbidding them their fat sandwiches on pain of death. As protest to this suppression of Jewish dietary laws, the sandwich itself became heroic, growing to mythic proportions, immense batonlike instruments of open war. Pastrami, legend tells, with one such sandwich felled a Cossack from his drunken horse. Right away both horse and rider were supposed to have been quietly salted down by the people of the village, and Pastrami fled. He was hot.

Nonetheless, attempts at demythologizing the Hero have produced various castrations, especially in the British Isles and Scandinavia. I refer here to the trimmed, crustless square, or tea sandwich, smeared with pastes and cress or cucumber slivers, and to the vulgar open-faced *Smörgås* where the meat lies raw and exposed in typically Swedish nudity. Sandwiches without their upper covering falsify the Reuben's orthodox origins. They are nothing but open-faced lies.

Unlike Rank, my loyal followers and I always preferred, therefore, the Sublimation Sandwich (see "Subs"). It is more psychological, less heroic, and a safer bet all around.

ERNEST JONES' WELSH OMELETTE

"Pour faire une Omelette il faut casser des oeufs."
—Letter to Fliess, 6 August 1899

What an irony of fate that it became Ernest Jones who was destined to write my biography. Jones! That little Welshman of all people! He couldn't even read my handwriting. Oh, yes, "undoubtedly a very interesting man," I once wrote, "but he gives me a feeling of, I was almost going to say, racial strangeness. He is a fanatic and doesn't eat enough. 'Let me have men about me that are fat', says Caesar. Jones always reminds me of the lean and hungry Cassius."

I paid my due to him in 1929 on the occasion of his fiftieth birthday, recalling his first paper at the 1908 Salzburg Congress. That paper, "Rationalization in Everyday Life," gives the clue to the entire subsequent misfortune of his biographical enterprise—the "standard" biography, like the "standard" edition. How typical of Jones to rationalize my discoveries into something standard: his own need to mask the racial strangeness of a native Welshman in British respectability.

And what a price he paid for acting out his sexual partial drives: in 1906, charged with indecent assault on two young girls; in 1908, a similar episode with a young hysteric, leading to his discharge from a London hospital; in 1911, blackmailed (he paid $500) by a patient in Toronto who said he had sex with her.◆

Clearly, that three-volume biography, written by one whose underdeveloped taste for food was compensated by overdeveloped taste for sex, has misrepresented my actual contributions to unraveling the libidinal mysteries of the psychical apparatus. The correct formula has always been: Libido = Appetite.

I say "native" in that Jones was, of course, Welsh; but not "native" in the meaning of original, inasmuch as my own attempts at ham omelette were recorded long before his, e.g., already in my letters to Fliess. Did Fliess leak this recipe to Jones? I had to inquire of Fliess directly: "You have said nothing about my Hamlet" (this was but an abbreviated way I had of referring to such recipes lest outsiders learn too readily what we were really writing about). "As I have not said anything about it to anyone else, I should be glad to have some short comment from you. Last year you turned down a number of my ideas with good reason."

While many cooks require special omelette pans of steel, iron, or aluminum, Jones never washed his own (cast-iron, of course, like his mind), only wiping it occasionally with a little oil. (He would have called such a prac-

---

◆ Freud seems unduly severe with these charges, especially in the light of Jones' own assiduously documented defense of himself in his autobiography, *Free Associations*. In the interest of fair play, we call the reader's attention to that work.—*The Editors*.

tice the "standard" way of making omelettes.) Even when he would visit us in London at that draughty Maresfield Gardens, the house he found for us, he never used to wash the pan after making his omelettes. I said nothing about this.

> Just as the 3 gently beaten eggs begin to set over medium heat, add the following filling: combine 2 tbs. chopped ham, 1 tbs. grated sharp English cheddar, and 1 tbs. chopped chives. Roll into omelette and roll omelette onto plate. Top with a grating of fresh black pepper.

NOTES
"He couldn't even read my handwriting."; Jones, *Life and Work*, vol. 2, p. 69 and p. 448. Also, letter to Jones, 20 November 1926.
"In 1906, charged"; *Journal of History of Behavioral Sciences*, vol. XVII (18 October 1981), p. 4.
"You have said nothing about my Hamlet. . . ."; letter to Fliess, 5 November 1897.

ALFRED ADLER'S SHORTCAKE

I agreed with Jung about Adler's work: it was totally without psychology. Adler could not bring any subtlety or refinement into things, substituting for the more complex and intriguing, the ready-made and simplistic. It is as if Adler were insisting that good cakes depended only upon their rising to the top, or that every cake fears falling flat.

> Mix together 2 cups flour, 3 tsp. baking powder, a slapdash of salt, 3 tbs. sugar. Blend in 1/2 cup butter, 1 beaten egg (see "An Egg Is Being Beaten"), and 1/3

cup milk (or be creative and use cream but then you will not be an Adlerian). Shape the cake any way you want (Adler's were always square). Place it in a greased cake pan. Bake at 450° for just 15 minutes or until done. (These so-called disciples of mine, always in a hurry, always looking for shortcuts, even with shortcake. I suppose today even the 15 minutes in this recipe may seem too much for some. Buy a ready-made shortcake mix then, and bake that. Adlerians could not tell the difference anyway.)

THE *DÉJÀ VUE* JAR

This small transparent box or jar may be made of plastic or glass. Its top fits securely. In it analysts keep little bits left over from the lovely meal they have just eaten (*Tagesreste*) and which they feel unable to throw into the maw of the disposal or the garbage sack. Instead, we place them in a *déjà vue,* on a shelf near the light in the refrigerator, where one can revisit them each time one opens the door. After one week, throw the contents out, and wash the *déjà vue* jar for further remnants. I am not suggesting that one ever eat anything from the *déjà vue* jar— that would only lead to intense fantasies of *fausse reconnaissance,* and perhaps even a chronic condition of *déjà vue* with a host of hideous complications (perennial consumption of leftovers, the inability to eat the freshest fruit or lettuce until last week's is consumed, etc.).

HERBERT SILBERER'S SILVER SHERBET

Herbert Silberer was the first among our faithful group to investigate the symbolism of alchemy (a priority only grudgingly granted by Jung). He later claimed to have invented this dish while experimenting alchemically with silver. Be that as it may, in 1909 when I first encountered this Silver Sherbet (hoping but to soothe my palate), Herbert was, as I described him then, only "an unknown young man, an upper-class degenerate whose father was a well-known member of the city council and an 'operator.' "

Poor Herbert, who would have expected his untimely suicide? Did he try too hard to please this surrogate father with trifles such as these? Or was it a more latent attempt at parricide? In any event, after eating this sherbet, I can assure you, your mouth will never be the same.

Combine 2 cups Pernod (ordinary anisette will not turn silver with ice), 2 cups water, and 1 cup granulated sugar in saucepan. Bring to boil over moderate heat, stirring constantly with the attention of an alchemist. Cool to room temperature. Pour into trays and set in freezer for several hours.

NOTE
"an unknown young man"; *The Freud/Jung Letters,* p. 242.

THE SCHREBER CAKE

Among my Cake Histories, one had an exceptionally long title: "Psycho-Analytic Notes upon an Autobiographical Account of a Case of Paranoia (Dementia Paranoides)," and so it is usually just called "The Schreber Cake."

An eminent Dresden judge, Daniel Paul Schreber, suffered a little breakdown in 1884 that lasted barely over a year. He wrote in revealing detail about all the paranoid delusions that assailed him while he was in the asylum. His book is called *Memoirs of a Neurotic.*

My study of Schreber was the first major attempt to

analyze what goes on inside a paranoid cake. I found the secret lies in repressed feelings about being a woman. Schreber had always been very correct, even ascetic; during his delusions, however, he found that he loved himself as a woman, especially his *Hausfrau*-like breasts, and that he could not stay out of the kitchen. *"Kinder, Küche, Kirche"*—children, kitchen, church—of course was the prescribed formula for a woman's life in the Germany of his day. Mixing flour and milk, good country eggs and butter, stirring the batter, and at last "having one in the oven"—that cured him.

Men, when you feel persecuted, when strange hatreds come into your mind, or when you are just tired of being men, drop whatever you are doing and go home at once, put on an apron and baker's hat, and make your Schreber Cake.

> Mix 1¹/₂ sticks butter, 1 cup sugar, 3 eggs, 1 tsp. baking powder, 1 lb. flour, ¹/₂ cup milk. Pour into greased tin and bake until brown. A few spoons of almonds, raisins, or other chopped fruit may be added to above mixture, but the true Schreber Cake, while at first sight appearing to be a fruitcake, has nothing inside it at all.

HANNS SACHSERTORTE

Hanns Sachs, a lawyer, joined our Vienna Society in 1910 and together with Otto Rank coedited *Imago* so that we might all have something to read while we ate our Sub Sandwiches. Later he became one of the small intimate circle, or Committee, of trustworthy colleagues who kept psychoanalysis going after so many defections. Sachs opened his own practice in Berlin, but soon moved to Boston. He was so sweet that more aggressive members of the circle, like Jung, used to refer to him as a piece of cake. Of that, I do not know; he was loyal. But certainly his Sachsertorte is much easier to make than the way I have observed them do it at our Hotel Sacher.

> Beat together 1 stick butter melted, $1/2$ cup sugar, $1/2$ cup flour, 4 egg yolks, 5 oz. melted chocolate, and 4 previously beaten egg whites. Pour into two greased baking pans. Bake in 325° oven until brown and tested with a knife that comes out clean. Cool on rack. Ice bottom layer with apricot jam, and top with Wish-Fulfillment Icing.

THE ANAL RETAINER

Ordinary colanders of enamel, metal, or plastic are all punched full of holes for quick rinsing of vegetables, draining salads, or for holding pasta under cold water to stop its softening. But sometimes one requires a retainer that bears the essential traits of the anal character—orderliness, frugality, obstinacy—to do the job. This colander has a single hole in its bottom, keeping back what would otherwise easily flow away. If you worry about your water bill or about all that good waste going down the drain, an anal retainer will give you a very pleasant feeling of control.

TOTEM AND TAPIOCA

The hatred of children for slippery food knows no bounds. The skim on hot cocoa, overcooked porridge, the sight of a parent swallowing an oyster, the slime of overboiled cabbage leaves or rhubarb can bring on intense loathing and revulsion. From this we are able to derive the loathing for slimy creatures in the Bible, for the toad and frog in fairy tales, and later perversions of the sexual drive. Among this class of loathed object belongs the innocuous dessert tapioca, so that when served together with the paternal injunction, "Eat what's on your plate!," a strong patricidal urge appears together with the pudding.

From this experience, encountered at my own supper table with my sons, and reported in the consulting room by patients of tapioca-eating families, I devised, in 1911 and 1912, my totem theory of prehistorical culture and primitive beliefs: "The old man of the horde" is killed by his sons and eaten—usually stewed, with tapioca on the side (the round pellets coming originally from the starch of the cassava plant of the primeval tropics, regions long known as the habitat of cannibals). The clan father is commemorated afterward by his sons as the totem animal of the tribe and revered, out of guilt, in ritual celebrations. (All those banquets: chicken à la King, mashed potatoes, or segmented grapefruit halves—all dishes featuring dismemberment, and representing in symbolic form primordial cannibalism. I knew what they were trying to say! The relevance to the Christian practice of eating the Host is too evident to dwell upon; see "Wonderbread, or the Future of an Illusion.")

While struggling with the slippery difficulties of my book *Totem and Taboo*—"the most daring enterprise I ever ventured," as I said in a letter—the gelatinous consistency of tapioca was unconsciously affecting the work. I felt "things boiling in my head" and spoke of the essay as a "beastly business" that "is not yet shaped in definite form." Reading the anthropological research that supported my ideas was like "gliding in a gondola," while my own thoughts had to "slither their way through." The reader will see how much I had tapioca on the brain.

My theory of totemism, I hasten to point out, did not prove true in the large Freud clan that I physically sired, my family having been fond and faithful. Soon enough, however, I found myself becoming a totem for people called "Freudians," my true clan perhaps, as they set about cannibalizing my work. I understand, too, that I am nothing but tapioca for non-Freudians, who abhor such ideas as too slippery. I can only conclude that these behaviors on the part of learned and respectable professionals can be explained by their early childhood experiences with squishy puddings.

> Here is one that is not so squishy. In the top of your Double-Bleuler, scald 2 cups milk. Add 2 tbs. tapioca and cook 10 minutes. Beat an egg yolk with 2 tbs. maple syrup and stir into tapioca mixture; cook until thickened. Chill. Beat an egg white stiff, adding 2 tbs. sugar. Fold into tapioca before serving. Serve with maple syrup and nuts on top.

FRAU LOU'S SALOMÉ PLATTER

Few women, maybe no others, have so captured my heart, and even my head, as Lou Salomé. (I do not refer to her by married name, Andreas-Salomé. Can one take that marriage seriously, after her affairs with Nietzsche, Rilke, Paul Rée, Poul Bjerre, and Victor Tausk? Besides, she never slept with that husband.) I have made it quite clear that though I was deeply attached to her, consulting with her intimately about my daughter Anna's ties with me, my feeling for Lou, as I have stated, "was without a trace of sexual attraction." Gossips, and they seem legion in my profession, have wondered why I—then nearing sixty—sent her roses, walked her home at 2:30 in the morning, and was crestfallen when she did not appear at a lecture.

The reason, I will tell it now, was her superb cuisine! We had so many secret recipes to exchange! You have seen her pictures—indeed, an *appetitliche Frau,* a wide-hipped, well-upholstered beauty, who surely knew what to eat. Of course she was too much for Nietzsche, poor mad devil, and for skinny neurasthenic Rilke, to say nothing of Paul Rée (the author of a dull book on moral sentiments) and Victor Tausk, who both killed themselves. I, alone, could appreciate this *femme fatale* because I, alone, knew her appetite for life was a life for appetite.

> Arrange a plate of olives, salami, tomatoes, and a few anchovies. Pour a light olive oil over it. Serve with crusty Vienna bread. If, however, your meetings, like ours, require more than the *kleine* Lou platter (above), a large Lou platter can be prepared. This features cold cuts from all the countries in which Frau Lou was, shall we say, "intimate," including Swiss *Bündnerfleisch* (dried beef), *mortadella* (Italian bologna), Tiroler cooked sausage (for Rilke), German *Braunschweiger,* Danish salami, and an international assortment of onions, pickles, relishes, etc. The final decoration of the large Lou platter, however, must be made with bjerres. If you cannot get Swedish lingon bjerres, use black bjerres or even, if you dare, "blue" bjerres.

NOTE
Cf. Roazen, *Brother Animal, the Story of Freud and Tausk,* pp. 42–58.

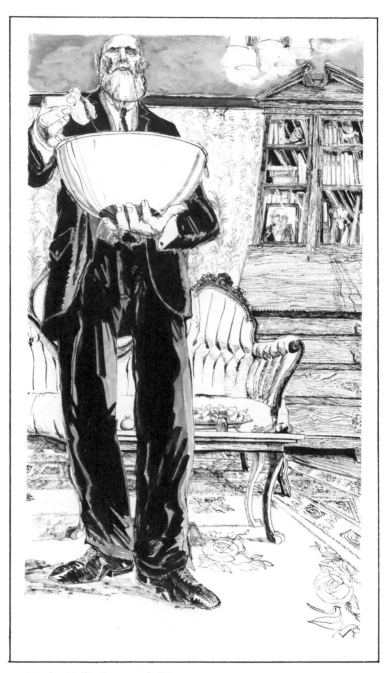

Stanley Hall's Guacamole Dip

VII.

FROM MY TRAVELS

Stanley Hall's Guacamole Dip, the *Zampóne* That Made Jung Faint, and Other Exotica

"America is already threatened by the black race. And it serves her right. A country without even wild strawberries."
—Freud to Marie Bonaparte, after visiting the United States. Quoted in *The Life and Work of Sigmund Freud,* vol. 2, Ernest Jones

A NOTE ON AMERICAN FOOD

"America is a mistake; a gigantic mistake, it is true, but nonetheless a mistake." That is what I told Ernest Jones after the trip that Jung, Ferenczi, and I took to Worcester, Massachusetts, in 1909 upon the invitation of G. Stanley Hall, the president of Clark University, to lecture there and be given honorary degrees, our first international recognition. But all those taco dips and chili dogs, potato chips and meatball grinders, *Himmel!* We spent our first day in New York at Coney Island and it was almost our last. That Brill! of all places to take us. I had dyspepsia literally for the rest of my life and I blamed it all on American cooking. I also had prostate trouble there; which was embarrassing, and the more so because Americans do not provide enough suitable places to relieve oneself. "They escort you along miles of corridors," I told Jones, "and ultimately you are taken to the very basement where a marble palace awaits you, only just in time." I would advise the foreign visitor to watch what he eats and drinks there, and especially where he eats and drinks it.

NOTES
"America is a mistake"; Jones, *Life and Work,* vol. 2, p. 60.
"They escort you . . ."; ibid.

MRS. STANLEY HALL'S MUSHROOM DIP

Nonetheless, Mrs. Hall, knowing my love for mushrooms, made a wonderful little dip for me in her food processor. She finely chopped 1 cup of fresh mushrooms, sautéed them for a few minutes with ½ cup chopped scallions, then added a few tbs. of sherry,

a genteel splash of their own Worcester Sauce, and a
little salt and pepper. The pan was removed from the
heat and 3 or 4 tbs. of *crème fraîche* were quickly
stirred in. I ate a bowlful, served on something else
that I had never seen before called "crackers."

STANLEY HALL'S GUACAMOLE DIP

Stanley decided, however, that he could top the
aforesaid recipe, and put in the food processor the
flesh of a ripe peeled avocado, a small onion, a splash
of Worcester Sauce (used in everything at the Halls!),
an unpeeled tomato, salt and cayenne pepper, and
turned it on and off several times quickly.♦

    It looked, at first, like a typical American mess,
but by the time it was mixed with a few more tbs. of
their *crème fraîche* (they had made bowls of this in
advance) and served on those crunchy chips of theirs,
even Jung and Ferenczi were crying *¡Ole!* to Clark
University and its honorary degrees. For my part, I
found that a beer or two helped with this one, and
since I did not have to go into the Halls' basement for
relief (their "marble palace" being on the second
floor), it was quite tolerable.

♦ No recipe for "Stanley Hall's Worcester Sauce" has been found
in the manuscript of this book or elsewhere. Since Freud refers
to it in several places, we are convinced that it exists and has
been removed or borrowed. It is possible that the missing recipe is to be found in the Freud Archives, but scholars will not
be given access to these papers, in most cases, until the year
2102. We do not know what is in this recipe that it should be
kept from the public so long, but of course we respect the
wishes of those for whom it might prove embarrassing. Until
2102, one can use Tabasco or angostura bitters as a substitute.
—*The Editors.*

PUTNAM'S GRILLED FISH

To have a professor of neurology at Harvard as one of us was very satisfying. James J. Putnam, in 1906, published, in Morton Prince's *Journal of Abnormal Psychology,* the first article in English on psychoanalysis. (The Boston police, instigated by a public ever so squeamish on sexual matters, later threatened to shut the journal down and arrest Prince for publishing "obscenities.") To be a pioneer in psychoanalysis in America was certainly a brave role, since one was constantly subject to diatribes and abuse. Still, I have always taken a special interest in the fate of psychoanalysis in America, the only country where I ever lectured, at Clark University, before a public audience.

After the ceremonies on that occasion, Jung, Ferenczi, and I went on to Niagara Falls for a ride on the *Maid of the Mists,* and then to Putnam's camp in the Adirondacks near Lake Placid, where for four days we stayed in primitive huts in the wilderness, fishing, drinking, and listening to that crazy Jung sing German songs into the night over a campfire.

It was not always fun being around Jung. There was too much Swiss crudity. At the 1911 Weimar Congress, Jung made some rather coarse jokes which provided relief from the pompous discussions, but during one of these interludes, I turned to Jung and said, "Damn it, man! Did you just fart?" To which he replied, "Of course, do you think I *always* smell like this?"

I suffered all during this time from a mild case of appendicitis and from what I later used to call "my American colitis." I had a lot of trouble with "Konrad" (as I used to call my bowel). Still, the grub at Putnam's camp was good, considering it was American. I was particularly interested in the way Putnam prepared fish.

He took a couple of pounds of striped bass fillets, and marinated them for an hour in a combination of oil, salt and pepper, and a handful of chopped fresh tarragon. The fish were then Charcot-Broiled for several minutes on both sides until they flaked easily when pierced with a fork. He served them on a bed of Boston lettuce and topped the fish with a few fresh tarragon leaves and melted butter.

NOTE

"Did you just fart?"; R. Steadman, *Sigmund Freud* (Middlesex: Penguin Books, 1982), p. 95.

MORTON PRINCE'S SPANISH RICE

Prince developed this recipe while writing his notorious personal attack on Theodore Roosevelt, the American president. He took the liberty of using psychoanalysis for this purpose, a practice I do not in the least condone, although some of my enemies have accused me of the same for my little study of Woodrow Wilson. The recipe, furthermore, is overdetermined, in my opinion, and one should not try to make it by himself; rather, one should obtain the assistance of helpers to put it all together. I do not believe, because of his claims for multiple personalities, that Prince ever made this by himself. When we would ask him, as he came bolting out of the kitchen to serve this dish at our psychoanalytic congresses, Did you really make this by yourself, Morton? he would always say yes, speaking softly.

Cook 1 cup white rice until tender. Meanwhile sauté for several minutes 1 large chopped onion, 1 chopped green pepper, a bullet of garlic minced, a big stick of chopped celery, and a helmet of sliced mushrooms. On still another burner in a large skillet, cook up several ounces of a good chopped sausage (not ground beef or any fashionable substitute like veal: Be a Rough Rider! Prince used to insist).

Add 2 or 3 chopped, seeded tomatoes and ¼ cup of diced pimientos to the sausage. Simmer, covered, for a few minutes. Keep checking all three pots constantly to make sure nothing is burning. Do not say, "I only have two hands!"—Think of Prince and his multiple personalities! Now add the onion mixture to the sausage mixture and both into the cooked rice. Add salt, pepper, a rifle blast of cayenne (Bully!) and a few tbs. of finely grated Sardo cheese (Parmesan type). Pour the entire batch into a buttered casserole. Top with more grated Sardo and bake, uncovered, for 20 minutes in 375° oven.

THE *ZAMPÓNE* THAT MADE JUNG FAINT

My views of Jung have been sufficiently amplified elsewhere (see "Jung Food"); here I wish only to offer the reader my own theory of Jung's fainting spells. Since he has taken the liberty of publicly discussing my own fainting spells, especially the time I fainted just prior to our trip to America in 1909, justice requires that we reciprocate.

Though he often fainted as a child, the most telling instance of this condition in the mature Jung was surely the occasion when, after a lifetime of intending to visit Rome but always putting it off, he finally went to the railroad station in Zurich, that bastion of Swiss Protestantism, and, while purchasing the long-anticipated tickets, with all that they promised, he fainted.

I had once formed an elaborate explanation of Jung's swooning based on his abstemious religious background (his avowed penchant for ancient polytheism notwithstanding) and its unconscious revulsion at the possibility of truly encountering the corruption and decay of contemporary Catholic Rome. Nonetheless, based on my own visits to Italy, I now think of poor Jung's hysterical faints with more sympathy. It is quite possible that these episodes were brought on merely by the contemplation of certain Italian dishes that may have been suggested to him. How he came to hear of them, I do not know; perhaps through one of his telepathic ("precognitive") dreams. I give them to the reader only in the interests of pathology, Italy's if not Jung's.

ZAMPÓNE WITH LENTILS AND BEANS

Zampóne looks like a spicy dish of pig's feet, but is actually part of the pig's intestines shaped like pig's feet. In Bologna it is formed like a ball but in Rome it is always sculpted like pig's feet (another version of it, called cotechino, is molded like a phallus, but I doubt that Jung or his circle would have had much interest in that dish, so drearily averse was he to sexual interpretations). With a needle, the pig's intestine is punctured in order not to explode while cooking. It is then put in cold water to cover and cooked over low heat for 5 hours, long enough to thoroughly remove the fat. The dish is served with lentils and beans which are cooked separately with sage and garlic.

The Italians say that if you eat this dish with lentils on New Year's Day it brings you money. That alone is an idea offensive to the Swiss, except as an explanation of Italy's condition.

LAMPREDOTTO

Another uncivilized dish that always guarantees gasps
from the northern European tourist is this recipe for
an Italian "sandwich." Tripe, or *trippa,* which is the
stomach of a cow, is boiled with a few chopped carrots
and tomatoes. The *lampredotto* is then wrapped in
newspapers for serving, and the water it was cooked in
poured over it for sauce. Even if it came wrapped in
his *Neue Zürcher Zeitung,* however, I doubt Jung
could have stomached this one (anymore than I could
stomach his tripology—all that tripe about extraverts
and introverts).

FÉGATO LARDELLATO

Feeling faint? If not, try this dish. Take a whole liver
of veal and lard the middle of it along with rosemary,
garlic, salt, and pepper. Wrap the liver in cabbage
leaves and place a slice of lard between the liver and
the leaves. Cook the *fégato lardellato* in a Double-
Bleuler for 5 or 6 hours (the odor of the cabbage
cooking is particularly foul and sure to get you if
nothing else). Meanwhile, cover several small white
onions in a pan of red wine and cook slowly for several
hours until the onions are reduced to a cream. When
ready, cut the liver into slices and cover with the
onion cream. *Buon appetito!*

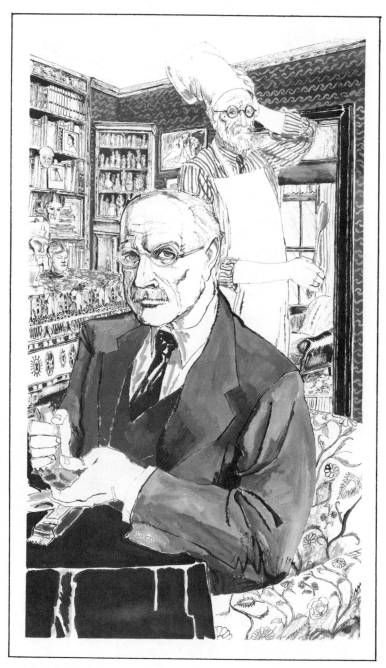

Jung Food

VIII.

THE LOYAL AND THE DISLOYAL

Jung Food and Tausked Salad, but also Ferenczi Fritters, and *Poires Belle* Helene Deutsch

"My enemies would be willing to see me starve. . . ."
—Freud at the Second International Psycho-Analytical Congress, Nuremberg, 1910. Quoted in *The Life and Work of Sigmund Freud,* vol. 2, Ernest Jones

What did cause the break with Jung? The passing years have given enough occasions, if not the leisure, for analyzing my relations with Jung. One by one I have gone through our differences—in age, in religion, in background, in temperament and ideas. But as much bound us together as separated us. Only by applying the psychoanalytic method, going back over the case history itself, incident by incident, did I come to find the true culprit: it was Ludwig Binswanger's buns, baked for me, and not for Jung, on that fateful Whitsun weekend in 1912 when I came to Switzerland—to Kreuzlingen to see him and not to Küsnacht to see Jung.

Why did not Binswanger invite Jung up for the weekend too? Of course, Jung demurred at coming uninvited, and I could not invite him to another man's house. But why did Binswanger let it occur, or shall I say arrange it, so that each of us, Jung and I, ended up accusing each other, and neither thought to blame Binswanger?

Memory, never trustworthy, yet nonetheless that mother of musing to whom psychoanalysis must always pay homage, recollects now, like Proust's madeleines, the special Whitsun buns, with a little cross engraved into them, that Binswanger brought hot from his oven to the Sunday breakfast table that morning.

Just enough for two, he said.

Had he run out of flour? Was there something between him and his wife that she had not gone to the store before closing? Was it the strict Swiss closing hours on the eve of holidays? Did he already know on Friday that there was "just enough for two"? Could he not have made more buns had he made them smaller? But most important of all, why were only Jung and I estranged after this episode and not Binswanger, too?

Reader, Binswanger's buns were curiously oversized, and doughy in the middle. I make them smaller, and with a double cross, in memory of the Kreuzlingen incident that led within a few weeks to the abrupt ending of my relationship with Carl Gustav Jung.

Dissolve 1 tbs. sugar and 1 tbs. yeast in 2 tbs. warm water. Combine with 1 cup scalded milk, 1/4 cup butter, 2 tbs. sugar, dash salt. Add 1 beaten egg (see "An Egg Is Being Beaten"), 1/2 cup raisins, 2 tbs. grated lemon rind, dash of cinnamon, and 2 to 3 cups flour (enough to keep batter moist). Let rise, covered, for 2 hours. Shape little dough balls on greased baking pan. Brush with egg white and let rise again, covered, for 1 hour. Bake in 425° oven for 25 minutes. Cool. With confectioner's icing, make a double cross on each bun.

VEAL OSKAR PFISTER

I could always count on the tolerance of the Reverend Oskar Pfister, a Swiss clergyman, toward this "unrepentant heretic," as I used to describe myself to him. He ever insisted that I was "a true Christian"; I would have to say the same for him, prey as he was to so much abuse in Zurich for his loyal defense of my views.

He was probably incautious in naming this veal dish after himself, and for daring to evoke that classic veal dish with one of his own so much more worldly, uncheeselike, and "Protestant." Yet for me, always, his will be the true "Veal Oskar."

Season a 3- or 4-lb. rump of veal with salt, pepper, and tarragon. Brown the roast in butter for several

minutes in a deep skillet over high heat. Add ¹/₂ cup
French white vermouth and ¹/₂ cup beef bouillon. Top
with a pfisterful of fresh tarragon, and simmer over
low heat for 2 hours, basting occasionally. Meanwhile,
sauté a pound of small white onions after sprinkling
them with a few tbs. flour and paprika. Several
minutes before roast is done, add the onions to the
roasting pan. Surround the roast on a platter with the
onions, and serve with the sauce, which you have
thickened with a little cream.

GROSS-FATHER POT-AU-FEU WITH BISMARCK SAUCE

On Gross of Graz, Jung was right: it was a pity he was such
a psychopath, since he was a keen supporter of my ideas.
He had even tried to reconcile my work with Kraepelin's,
in whose clinic he once worked as an assistant. (At one
point, though, he had to be forcefully restrained, by none
other than Jones, from taking Kraepelin to court: Gross
wanted to demonstrate that Kraepelin, who detested psychoanalysis, was simply ignorant of it—Gross thought
such ignorance a crime.) I once believed only he and Jung
would ever make original contributions to our subject, and
time, I think, has proved me correct. But what contributions!

Eventually addicted to opium, he also suffered from
toxic cocaine paranoia (but his real problem was his
father). Jung, on my advice, had Gross committed, and
worked him through the withdrawal period with the understanding that I would then do an analysis; my self-de-
fense mechanism, however, nicely prevented me from
that, and Jung did the analysis himself. Whenever he got
stuck, he said, Gross analyzed him! (It is surely from Gross'

book, *The Secondary Function of the Brain,* that Jung got his introvert–extravert theory, so Jung should stop his kvetching.)

While all went very promisingly at first, Gross suddenly jumped over the garden wall and escaped. It was all downhill from there, leading to his death several years later in Berlin from, I shudder to say it in a cookbook, starvation.

Otto Gross' own therapy was orgiastic. He called it the Cult of Astarte, his Babylon being a polymorphous perverse response to the sexual tyranny of Judaeo-Christian monogamy. This was a neat way of getting back at his father.

The original sin, Otto said, was the enslavement of women. Thus he set about forming sexual liaisons with some of the most interesting and unenslaved women of his day, including Frieda von Richtofen, who later married D. H. Lawrence.

Orthodox analysts finally could stand it no longer when, in the anarchist colony of Ascona, Switzerland, he rented a barn for narcotic and sexual orgies, in which people were urged to "act out" their repressions. It was there that he gave poison to one of his mistresses, Sophie Benz, and she voluntarily killed herself, no doubt as part of her self-emancipation.

Otto fled to Berlin, where his father, a famous criminologist and magistrate of Bismarck's generation and temperament, had him arrested as a degenerate and dangerous psychopath (showing the police a certificate to that effect that he had obtained from C. G. Jung). Poor Otto said the arrest was in retaliation for an essay he wrote on sadism in which he had used his father as an example.

The arrest became a sensation in the anarchist press of that time, and Otto became a hero, a legend, one might say. "Free Otto Gross!" became the cry of thousands who shared his revolutionary call for the liquidation of the patriarchalist family and its bourgeois sexuality. (Gross' followers later organized the Dada movement in Berlin with much the same purpose.)

As a result of the protests, he was freed on condition that he enter analysis with Stekel. But this did not last long, and he fled to Prague, where he became an influence on that very strange writer, Franz Kafka, who declared himself ready to join Gross in a battle against the world's fathers.

When I reflect on what havoc I have wrought on my fellow fathers of this world, who, it must be said, rarely ask more of life than to hear that cherished term of endearment, "Papa," uttered now and then on the lips of their beloved brood as they all sit down to a good dinner, it is enough to give me pause. (I recall now, too, Otto once telling me that his earliest recollection was of his father warning a visitor about him, "Watch out, he bites." Considering his death, it would appear that he did not bite enough.)

I recount this long, sad story of Otto Gross only to explain the curious, and for me at least, quite hearty, dish that follows. Otto was a vegetarian, which follows from his pro-matriarchal taste; a contempt for the father is often behind this aberration. But he was also anti-wine, and this seems to me the fly in his ointment, the broken linchpin in his matriarchal machine, the goo in his goulash. He did not understand that only Dionysus can defeat the patriarchal Apollo. Perhaps for him cocaine was Dionysian ritual enough, a substitute for wine. Alas, I can attest that it is not. He should have realized, with his nostrils blown away, and with blood on his shirt collar from the Dionysian destruction of his nose, what was happening to him.

I suspect, therefore, that Otto never made this recipe for Gross-Father Pot-au-Feu, which he sent me once when I asked him how he managed to survive. Just the thought of eating this, he said, was enough to keep him going.

One is supposed to bring it to the table as if it were an ordinary pot-au-feu, spooning out the beef onto a dish, but then surprise! as the host digs deeper, he finds a sausage (and exclaims), and then a chunk of pork (and exclaims again), and then a chicken (here I stop exclaiming).

In a large cauldron of beef bouillon and chicken broth and water, simmer together, for several hours, a large piece of rumpsteak, a large hock of pork, a whole chicken, and a couple of pounds of German sausage, the bigger the better. Do not bother to trim the fat off the meat; it should be fat and Bismarckian. One should, however, truss the meat, I think, rather than let it all hang out. That would not be Bismarckian. Do not bother to add the meat at various times depending on how long each takes to cook: they all simmer together equally in Otto's recipe because they are all meat, and he would not make distinctions. (The sausage will get especially bloated.)

Every so often put into the pot a carrot or a single stalk of celery or a peeled onion. After an hour, as the meat goes on simmering, the vegetables will be destroyed. Remove the vegetables from the pot and throw it away or, if you prefer, keep these little reminders of Otto on a plate to be served to the astonishment of the meat-eaters after they have started eating. They will say, not recognizing the little fellows at all, What are those?

Add whatever seasonings will make the dish palatable for you. (Otto could never apparently find any; his recipe does not contain any.)

Meanwhile prepare a Bismarck Sauce: simmer 1 cup cream until reduced by half. In a bowl, beat together 1 tsp. French mustard with at least 3 tsp. German mustard, then beat in the cream. Add 1 tsp. of paprika for a nice red color.

Carve the meat, and top with sauce (parsley, that good old bourgeois herb, helps to cover everything up, if that is your disposition). Serve with a good

German red wine, if you can find one, such as a Kaiserstuhl, an Assmanshauser, or an Ahrweiler.

NOTE
"On Gross of Graz"; see especially Martin Green, *The Von Richtofen Sisters* (New York: Basic Books, 1974), pp. 32–47.

SAUCE NARCISSE

Sauté 2 tbs. minced onion in 2 tbs. butter for 5 minutes. Stir in 2 tbs. flour. Slowly add 1 cup hot beef stock (fish or chicken stock if you intend the sauce for those dishes). Keep stirring until smooth. Add desired salt and pepper and 2 tbs. of your favorite Scotch, bourbon, or cognac. Thicken sauce, if necessary, with more flour, but make sure it is smooth. Pour sauce into your Irma's Injector and, squeezing it carefully, write your name in bold letters over the roast, steak, fish, or chicken just before serving. You may even sign individual servings if you wish.

IRMA'S INJECTOR

In the famous dream of the night of July 23–24—the first dream I ever thoroughly interpreted with my new method—this piece of equipment appears as an unclean hypodermic syringe used to inject the patient Irma with a chemical solution to cure her of a diseased mouth. But I have only recently penetrated the dream's true disguise: Irma's injection was of course Irma's Injector, that marvelous squeezer she had invented for filling hollow pastries (long éclairs, cream puffs, *puits d'amour,* and *Krapfen* with their hidden spot of jelly). The canvas (or strong linen) bag holds the mixture to be inserted. The left hand keeps the bag closed and applies pressure, while the right hand inserts the metal or plastic nozzle into the shell to be stuffed. Irma's Injector, with a finer tip, can also be used for decorating cakes, scalloping edges of bright vegetable purees on plates of *nouvelle cuisine,* and for signing autographs (see "Sauce Narcisse"). It should not, however, be used for medical purposes.

BIRTH TRAUMA CAKE
(*Geburtstrauma Kuchen*)

Martha used to make this every sixth of May, my birthday, when the very first wild strawberries, our *Walderdbeeren,* began to appear in the Vienna woods. (But *Walderdbeeren* are not necessary—especially not for children for whom ordinary strawberries or cherries will do.)

The cake never actually bakes, though it believes it does and looks as if it has. It is put into a 450° oven which is then immediately shut off, providing a primordial shock to its little system that traumatizes it for the rest of its short life. Let it stay in the warmth of the oven to recuperate for several hours, gradually cooling to room temperature.

Beat 6 egg whites along with a smack of salt and a pinch of cream of tartar. Gently fold in 1½ cups sugar. When perky, almost able to stand up on its own, pour into a buttered springform pan and give it its shock in the oven. After it is born several hours later (or overnight) give it a good *Schlag* (see "The Interpretation of Creams") and top with the berries, a few of which may be crushed into a sauce that flows down from the top.

JUNG FOOD

Let me assure the reader that I neither eat Jung Food myself nor recommend it to anyone. The dishes mentioned below are included for the sake of an objective history of the psychoanalytic movement, but are not part of its culinary canon. When Jung broke away he took his food with him—and good riddance, a feeling which any sensible reader will share, I am certain.

In the first place, Jung Food is addictive, based largely on sweeteners. It is readily found and easily consumed, what Jung himself called "collective." Perhaps in Zurich it is different, but as far as I am concerned, what is readily found, consumed, and collected is nothing but garbage.

Jung Food comes wrapped in all those high-sounding names of gods, or "archetypes" as Jung would fancifully call them, but what they come down to, in real life, is nothing but zodiacal candy: Mars Bars, Milky Ways, and Twinkies. (The Americans, of course, are the worst offenders of all here, and the most devoted to Jung Food.) A particularly offensive example of Jung Food is something called Almond Joy, a cheap translation of the word for Jung's ever-present mandalas—*Mandel* being but the German word for almond—and of my name as well. It is as if Freud—joy—is to be granted, ever so grudgingly, this modest place in the Jungian vision.

Jung Food beverages—especially in their American manifestation—bear further witness to this sweetened and uplifting spirit. There, the drinks are effervescent with such names as Sprite, Mountain Dew, and Coke. Some even pretend to be medical, like Dr. Pepper.

In the second place, Jung Food has been strongly influenced by the East: Chop Sueys, I Chings, Orphic egg rolls, Egg Foo Jungs. This cultish esotericism, at bottom, is nothing but Sub Gum Moo Pan, loaded with MSG and disguised as a secret concoction of golden wisdom.

Most Jungian of all, perhaps, are fortune cookies, for Jung Food always carries concealed messages. Jung tried to dignify these cookie messages by coining the term "synchronicity," a password among food Jungies, to account for strange coincidences of fate, such as when you suddenly feel ill at a Chinese restaurant and your fortune cookie asks: "Botulism?" So striking a demonstration of the subtle interconnectedness of all things is what Jung tried to explain with synchronicity. What nonsense! Nowhere better than here does the contrast between his pseudo-science and my science of psychoanalysis with its tested hypotheses of the primal horde, infantile sexuality, and the origins of religion show more clearly.

In the third place, the Hindu influence makes Jung Food hot and exciting. Hot food favors the mouth, perhaps, but it leads the Jungies (those who curry favor with the Guru of Zurich) to neglect the nether orifice of the alimentary canal. "What goes in, must come out" is a lesson of nature that even the smallest child must learn. Burned by Jung Food, Jungies fail to recognize (do they even read?) our researches into anality. This failure causes severe depressive symptoms in advanced Jung Food addicts who then often come to Freudians for a second analysis. There they uncover the hidden meaning of analysis: anal-lysis, *lysis* being the Greek word for relaxing, loosening, softening.

Another effect of the Hindu influence is the fact that Jung Foods are usually stained yellow with saffron or turmeric, a yellow that will not wash off. Jung Food can permanently taint the hands and clothing of those with the habit. Jung tried to legitimize this yellowing with a fancy name he found in alchemy (*citrinitas*), and he also psychologized it by stating that yellow refers to the function of intuition. As I see it, however, it is Jung Food that turns

color, and as he jumped gently about, the vegetables acquired just enough of the oil to shine without being soggy.
Before this, I used to pour dressings over my salads, virtually drowning them in an oleaginous shower. From Viktor I saw that the dressing (he called it the "undressing")
goes first and the salad is "Tausked" just before one eats it.
(You do not, of course, have to use the floor, or even a bed
of lettuce; a large bowl is suitable for the purpose.)

Soon, however, the War laid claim to Viktor's services.
When he returned several years later, he was still the cute
little cucumber of our salad days. But I was now in my six-
ties, and wilting. I tried valiantly to oil up the old avoca-
does for another toss, but it was useless. The War had
soured all; there was simply too much vinegar in my vinai-
grette. (I even submitted to a rejuvenatory operation on
my testicles, the so-called Steinach operation, but to no
avail.)

Taking myself to Tausk in such a woeful state was out
of the question. I decided to arrange a liaison for him instead with a woman analyst five years his junior, that lus-
cious pear, Helene Deutsch. I thought a pear salad might
be a welcome change for him. She was in a training analysis with me at the time; I figured she would thus keep me
in touch with Tausk's leguminous fantasy life without my
having to concede to him the loss of my powers, and thus
my authority. Besides, I thought he would introduce her to
Tausked Salads, which would be useful in her later career.
I relied, as always, on his sense of the polymorphous perverse, or at least of noblesse oblige.

I found, however, that after a while she had less and
less to say of Tausk during her hour; all she wanted to discuss was dessert (see *"Poires Belle* Helene Deutsch"). This
led me to snooze: and when, twice, she caught me when
my cigar dropped to the floor, I decided I had had enough.
I told her that for her own good she would have to give up

either her analysis of Tausk or my analysis of her. To my horror, she chose to give up Tausk! Was it, I wondered, the endive? the uncomfortable bed of lettuce?

I must say I did not think Viktor would take the end of his analysis so seriously, or see it as rejection. There were so many women who still wanted him, including a rich Serbian aristocrat who even offered to buy him a professorship (the only way you get them here, as I can attest in my own case), but he refused, saying he did not care for *Srpski ajvar* (a Serbian vegetable caviar) and preferred his vegetables raw.

Within three months he was dead, with a noose around his neck and a gun in his hand, and for all I know covered in olive oil, too. He had sent me a nice suicide note and explained that he would not be able to attend, as usual, the Wednesday night meeting of our Vienna Society.

Naturally, I wrote a grand obituary for him in the journal: "Here was a man of importance," etc. But to Lou I wrote the truth: "I confess I do not really miss him." I had discovered, quite on my own, arugula.

NOTES
Roazen, *Brother Animal, the Story of Freud and Tausk:*
"Lou thought Tausk was my double . . . ," p. 63.
"a rejuvenating operation . . . ," p. 50.
"including a rich Serbian aristocrat . . . ," p. 106.
"twice she caught me when my cigar dropped . . . ," p. 96.
"He had sent me a nice suicide note . . . ," pp. 120–124.
"Here was a man of importance . . . ," cited p. 133.
"I confess I do not really miss him . . . ," cited p. 134.

THE *ANHANG*

More and more people are finding out that the English and American translations of my German terms have distorted some of my best recipes and spoiled many a dinner party. For instance, an *Anhang* is not a supplement or an addendum tacked on as an afterword. It refers to a row of hooks for hanging up basting spoons, prodding forks, long spatulas, and ladles. They do not belong in a drawer, out of sight and out of reach. An what can you hang them without an *Anhang?* Besides, a drawer takes two hands: one to pull it open and one to reach into it. I learned this sort of handiness during pathological dissections. As necessity is the mother of invention, so the morgue is the father of the kitchen.

GRODDECK'S PUREE OF WILDEBEEST

Georg Groddeck contributed the id to psychoanalysis. Considering his manner, I suggested he call it the odd, a more appropriate appelative. Groddeck was so odd, or should I say so id, that I readily took this term for the psyche's primitive layer of wild bodily appetites from him: tall, Samson-shouldered, but with a clean-shaven scalp, large ears, and crude.

At our solemn congress at The Hague in 1920, Groddeck leaped to the platform to announce to the assembled professionals, "I am a wild analyst."

Anna took offense.

—What an idiot! she exclaimed.

—What an Id, I said, but I found him endearing, and not without genius.

At his sanitorium in Baden-Baden, where he treated

Ferenczi and where he wanted to treat me, Groddeck propounded an idea of treatment that was daunting. "It is my practice," he wrote, "to kneel upon the patient's stomach and tell him to take deep breaths so as to press out the fluid contents of the viscera, the blood, and the lymph." All very well—but the case in question was a bedridden woman over seventy! It is of course an idée fixe among our critics that Freudians are overly reductive, but Groddeck was indeed reducing patients to puree.

Even more unforgivable was the fact that he mucked about with their food. Frau A. was given only a slice of bread, a bit of fruit, a cup of tea for breakfast; a sliver of steamed fish, boiled carrot, tea and a sweet wafer for lunch. While such "cuisine" will strike the average British palate—I know it now so well—as altogether toothsome, it was, from our viewpoint, debilitating.

Nor was this by any means the end of his medicine. He then ordered Frau A. to walk a mile a day; he might as well have insisted she jog it. *Hic labor, hoc opus,* and all that, but even in the *Aeneid* one would wince at seventy when an Id rises.

Sometimes Groddeck went to esophageal extremes, having a patient who could not eat certain foods without nausea fed exclusively on those foods. Clearly, he was repressing in his patients the very Id he feared in himself.

As for Groddeck's Puree of Wildebeest, the reader need have no fear of a gnu experience at the supermarket. At the Freud house, we use sweet potatoes instead. Bake 3 or 4 sweet potatoes in their skins in 350° oven for an hour. Scoop their flesh (you may kneel on them if you like) into a food processor with the juice of an orange, a little wild honey, salt and pepper. Process till smooth. It is guaranteed to soothe whatever savage beast you have.

NOTES

C. M. Grossman and S. Grossman, *The Wild Analyst* (London: Barrie and Rockcliff, 1965):
"I am a wild analyst . . . ," cited p. 48.
"It is my practice . . . ,"cited p. 49.

MARIE BONAPARTE'S BREAST OF CHICKEN
(*Suprème de volailles* Bonaparte)

Such strange, strong women around me. Lou Salomé, H.D., Helene Deutsch, Minna and Anna, and Paula who brought the food to our family table. Has the reader ever looked at the ladies in the front row of that classic picture of our 1911 Congress? What somber intensity! But could any of them cook?

Marie Bonaparte, my pupil, my confidante, and, not the least, my wealthy benefactress, was quite another cup of tea. Her picture in décolleté in the *Almanach* exhibits her soft shoulders and lovely white skin that I freely associate with this dish. As Princess George of Greece and living in Paris, nobody expected her to cook. But her tastes were odd: she was fascinated by incest, women murderers, and the servant problem, claiming to recall a coitus that went on in her presence between her nursemaid and her groom when she was not even one year old.

The Princess' main work was on Edgar Allan Poe and his melancholic drinking, though it is well established that drinkers never eat well, if at all. Absorbed as she was by the Parisian bedroom view of life, she never ventured to consider the culinary habits of savage peoples, so that when she analyzed the symbolism of horns and the cuckolded husband, she missed the whole point. Savages hunted horned animals to bring back trophies for the table, and they turned cocks into capons because they tasted better.

That reminds me: someday I must write on the symbolism of the raw and the cooked in primitive cultures.

Remove skin from chicken breast with your fingers. Disjoint the wing. Strike deep against the breastbone with your knife! Pound the thing a few times with your hand. Pull flesh off bone any way you can, but try to keep the meat in one piece. Remove wing. Keep the bones for chicken soup, in case of illness. You are now ready for Chicken Bonaparte.

Sauté a chopped onion in butter and a sprinkle of cinnamon. Brown the chicken breasts in the onions for several minutes, until tender. Remove to warm platter, leaving onions in pan. Pour a glass of Five Star Metaxa Brandy (pretend you are Princess George of Greece) into pan of onions. Boil for a few minutes. Add 1 cup cream and cook until slightly thickened. Pour sauce over chicken breasts, top with parsley and a royal soupçon of cinnamon.

NOTES

Cf. "Der Fall Lefebvre," *Imago* XV/I, 1929; "Der Tod Edgar Poes," *Almanach der Psychoanalyse* 1933, p. 224; Foto, *idem.;* Jones, *Life and Work,* vol. 3, p. 129; "Uber die Symbolik der Kopf trophaen," *Imago* XIV/I, 1928.

FERENCZI FRITTERS

Sandor, a loving, good man au fond—but dead before sixty. Alas, how many tributes, how many obituaries of men far younger than myself I have had to write. How each recipe brings back a face and a moment in the history of the psychoanalytic movement! Short as he was, Ferenczi made contributions to theory and practice that are head and shoulders above so much being written today. And if ever our correspondence were to be published, his place would be firmly recognized.

Sandor did not understand, however, the fundamental principle of all psychoanalysis (and of much cooking, too, I might add): abstention. In his later years—and this recipe stems from that time—he held the conviction that one could effect far more with one's patients if one gave them the love withheld from them as children. Hugging patients, holding them in one's lap—these physical gratifications of biological needs, according to Sandor, could lead to a ferenczied afternoon of therapeutic practice.

But how many patients could one shuffle on and off one's little lap each day? And the same patient five times a week? It must have been exhausting. When he actually started kissing patients, and allowing them to kiss him, I had to write him a word of warning: "Now picture what will be the result of publishing your technique. . . . A number of independent thinkers in matters of technique will say to themselves: why stop at a kiss? Certainly one gets further when one adopts 'pawing' as well, which after all doesn't make a baby. And then bolder ones will come along who will go further to peeping and showing—and soon we shall have accepted in the technique of analysis the whole repertoire of demiviergerie and petting parties, resulting in an enormous increase of interest in psychoanalysis among both analysts and patients."

But Sandor never would listen, even becoming indignant with me. And when I asked him once, in a conciliatory mood, if he had any interesting recipes, this strange mishmash is what he sent me from Budapest.

Mash 3 cups cooked eggplant. Beat ferencziedly into it 3 tbs. flour, 1 egg you have previously beaten (see "An Egg Is Being Beaten"), 1 finely minced red pepper, and 1 tsp. lemon juice. Keep beating mixture until you are beside yourself. Dash salt, pepper, cayenne, and nutmeg. Beat some more. Drop tablespoonfuls into hot, deep, smothering fat. Brown well. Dry fritters lovingly and gently with paper towels, and top each with a maternal sprinkling of paprika.

NOTES

"Now picture what will be the result . . ."; Jones, *Life and Work,* vol. 3, p. 164.

ABRAHAM'S KIDNEYS

My biblical interest in Abraham, unlike my fascination for Moses, produced no publishable work. Was it because in our circle I could easily become Moses, but there already was an Abraham? I refer, as the reader might surmise, to Karl Abraham of Berlin, loyal disciple to the end—and bizarre end it was, brought on prematurely in 1925 following his swallowing of a fish bone.

Is this the fate the gods have in store for one whose attention was focused so profoundly, and perhaps too narrowly, upon the anal? For it was Dr. Abraham's scientific contributions to the psychology of the anus that have placed us all forever in his debt.

I have named this recipe in his honor, remembering from my biblical and classical studies that the gods do not demand foods requiring too much attention. They do not extract fish bones, being perhaps too farsighted for the task. Rather, they delight in animal parts wrapped in delicate fat. As it says in Leviticus: "Two kidneys and the fat that is on them . . . is an offering made by fire, of sweet savour to the Lord."

Here, then, is a dish with no bones, and the slices in their light, fragrant fat slip down the throat harmlessly.

You must use a whole veal kidney, wrapped in its fat. Trim fat slightly to get a small football shape, but be careful not to cut into the kidney which lies buried, invisible, in the fat. If there is not enough fat, ask the butcher for more kidney fat and truss it. Salt and pepper liberally. Insert sprigs of rosemary. Place on rack (to let fat drip) in 400° oven for 15 minutes. Remove and add more fresh rosemary. Cook 10 to 15 minutes more. If you want the kidney done more than slightly pink, cook it longer but at reduced temperature (375°).

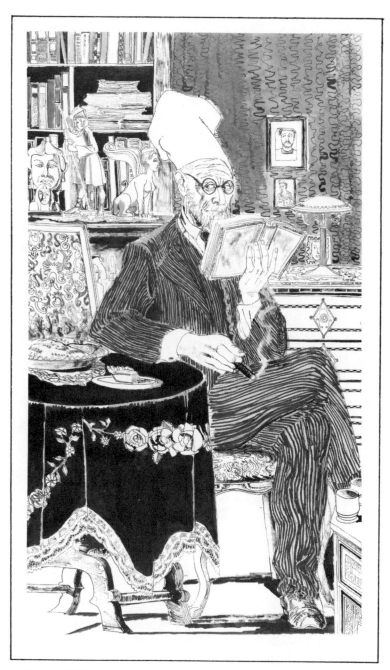

Paranoid Pie

IX.

EASY TO MAKE

Superegonog, Morning and Melon Dishes, Paranoid Pie

"The soup is on the table, else I should go on grumbling. . . ."
—Letter to Fliess, 16 September 1895, in *Letters of Sigmund Freud, 1873–1939,* ed. E. L. Freud

AN EGG IS BEING BEATEN

My 1919 paper traced the origin of sadomasochistic disorders to the early repression of the fantasy, "a child is being beaten." That paper with that title has received much not unjustified acclaim. The years have shown, however, that one must go back further than the beaten child, further even than the beating the newborn takes in the birth trauma, back to the beating of the very egg itself. From the fantasies surrounding the egg, psychoculinary development may go in several directions: identification with the beaten egg leads to masochism; identification with the beating of the egg leads to sadism; and if a person identifies with the egg-beater itself (whether fork, whisk, or rotary), to mechanisms of repression.

Since so much can go wrong at the very earliest stage of a recipe (*ab ovo*), it is crucial, when working with eggs, to watch out for fantasies. Keep to the ego's reality principle. Count out exactly the number of eggs needed. Crack them briskly. Make your separations distinctly when the recipe calls for them. Toss out the shells without an afterthought. Above all, do not identify (especially with egg shells). If you want to be a good cook, you must learn to separate the ego from the egg with one flick of the wrist.

SUPEREGONOG

A human life must find its way between the desirous drives of the id and the inhibiting injunctions of the superego. Our lives are but compromises and the instrument of this compromise we call the ego. The ego often renounces activities and wishes in order not to become involved in conflict with the superego (which affects the ego with feelings of guilt and anxiety). Rather than feel guilty we forgo the pleasure that would bring on the guilt. The ego, then, lives a life of quiet indigestion, a plain man's life of plain food. Therefore, a good deal of the culinary art is directed toward allaying anxiety attacks and guilt feelings by removing the inhibitory effect of the superego. Nothing in my experience aids this supportive therapy of the ego, by softening the strictures of the superego, more than the age-old *pharmakon:* fermented or distilled spirits.

> First pour a generous cup of rum into a bowl. In separate bowl, beat to a ferenczi 6 egg yolks, $^1/_4$ cup sugar, $1^1/_2$ cups milk, 6 already beaten egg whites (see "An Egg Is Being Beaten"), 1 cup whipped cream, and a careful grating of fresh nutmeg. Chill. When ready to serve, remove Superegonog from the refrigerator, and pour the bowl of rum back into the bottle.

MORNING AND MELON

Breakfast commemorates humanity's step out of the bedroom, from the long starvation of sleep, to the upright posture at the counter laden with beverages, grains, sweets, eggs, fruits, and the newspaper. What should be a cheerful moment recapitulating the history of the race from its predawn origins, becomes for neurotics a time of mourning over last night and melancholia regarding the day ahead. As I said in my 1917 essay, "Mourning and Melancholia," married pairs neurotically enact "countless conflicts in which love and hate wrestle together for the object; the one seeks to detach the libido from the object, the other to uphold [it] against assault."

I should have been more explicit in this article and pointed out that by lididinal object I meant the morning melon (though grapefruit, papaya, or even apple Danish can be the fruit of desire at this time). These libidinal wrestling matches make for a mournful morning, and may bruise the melon or worse. As a precaution against such breakfast imbroglios, I used to advise my patients, particularly those whose analytical hours were scheduled before 10 A.M. (and who were thus especially afflicted with morning melancholia), to cut a slice of ripe honeydew into spoonsize wedges and sprinkle them with ginger; some were merely told to put cinnamon over their broiled grapefruit; others advised to squeeze a fresh lime over papaya halves. Such simple touches, but you will be surprised at how they can cut down, after a while, on analyst fees.

NOTE
"countless conflicts . . ."; "Mourning and Melancholia," in *Coll. Papers IV* (London: Hogarth Press, 1925), p. 168.

ON CHICKEN RECIPES

Tell it not in Gath, publish it not in the streets of Askelon, in the land of the Philistines, but I do not like chicken. Why do I not like chicken? How I have pondered this! The sexual interpretation comes all too easily to the analyzed mind: chick, *poule, altes Huhn*—all terms of contempt for women. Thus, eating chicken—the breasts, the thighs, the-part-that-goes-over-the-fence-last—becomes all too evident: it is the kind of facile interpretation we get nowadays from graduates of psychoanalytical institutes, some of which, *horribile dictu,* bear my name.

More likely the sources of my chicken phobia can be found in infantile reminiscences of Jewish stories told in

Moravia where I was born and where it was said: When a poor Jew eats a chicken, one of them is sick.

In our household, Martha served chicken only when we entertained guests, whose gabble at table interfered with my concentration and forced this unwelcome food upon me. Should I forsake the dinner and retreat to my writing table, or satisfy my needs for family life and eat the accursed bird, swallowing my anxiety with it?

This tormenting dilemma I disguised in the form of an anecdote in a letter to Fliess: "A husband and wife decided to have chicken for a festival dinner, but could not decide whether to kill the cock or the hen; so they consulted the Rabbi: 'Rabbi, what are we to do, we've only one cock and one hen. If we kill the cock, the hen will pine, and if we kill the hen, the cock will pine. But we want to have a chicken dinner for the festival. Rabbi, what are we to do?' 'Kill the cock,' the Rabbi said. 'But then the hen will pine.' 'Yes, that's true; so kill the hen.' 'But Rabbi, then the cock will pine.' 'Let it pine,' said the Rabbi."

Rabbis and sick chicken jokes, enough already! When I'm eating, I'm eating, and free association must stop. The work of the couch is not the work of the table.

Nonetheless, I have included here several chicken recipes gathered from associates and patients who played important roles in my life. Despite personal bias against the fowl itself, I offer such recipes to the reader in the spirit of truth, science, and completeness.

NOTE
"A husband and wife . . ."; letter to Fliess, 28 May 1899.

CIPOLLA DI POLLO ASCHAFFENBURG

I once swore to myself that if Gustav Aschaffenburg ever came to our house for dinner, this dish, which I observed being prepared once in a trattoria in Siena, would be served. The reader will think ours was the House of Atreus, but there was little chance, of course, of Aschaffenburg ever being invited. (Still, my own distaste for chicken makes me shudder even now and wonder how even my intense antipathy for this minor professor of psychiatry at Heidelberg could have led me to such distasteful schemes—but *Nemo me impune lacessit,* I always said.)

Aside from his personal unpleasantness, his attacks on me were motivated by the fact that he could not stomach sexuality, "that troublesome factor so unwelcome in good society," as I once wrote Jung about him.

Here is the recipe: just take the stomach of a chicken (reach down there!) and fry it whole with onions.

NOTE
"that troublesome factor . . ."; *The Freud/Jung Letters,* 3F, ed. William McGuire.

THE WOLFMAN'S EASY WALNUT CHICKEN

My most famous case—I wish I could say my most famous recipe too but Freud Clams is surely that, the way Americans eat them—was of a young Russian aristocrat, Sergius Pankejeff. I diagnosed the patient as being "completely dependent upon other people and entirely incapacitated." It did not occur to me then—this was before the Great War— that this diagnosis fits all aristocrats.

Nonetheless, his dreams were interesting, especially the one where he lay in bed looking out the window onto a big walnut tree on which six or seven white wolves sat staring at him as if ready to eat him up. (Rank, whose imagination always tended too much toward the literal, reduced the wolves to the photographs of the six members of the Committee on my consulting room wall.) Through further analysis I was able to determine that the white wolves really stood for his parents' white underwear.

I was never quite successful with the Wolfman. He came back for further analysis with me after the War—and to borrow money, which I gladly loaned him. In fact, he spent the rest of his life in analysis with my successors, making a living for himself as an insurance man and as Freud's most famous case.

Yet I was able to get him over the fear of those wolves eating him. I simply asked him what he thought the wolves would rather eat if they could not have him. Then, together, we devised the following recipe. Composing it was distasteful for me, because of my loathing for chicken. Nonetheless, an analyst is always in service of his patient.

Cut up chicken and brown in butter. Cover with boiled chicken stock and 1 cup vodka. Simmer for 30 minutes. Add a pound of chopped walnuts and continue cooking 15 minutes. Serve cold.

NOTES

"I diagnosed the patient . . ."; Karin Obholzer, *The Wolfman, Conversations with Freud's Patient Sixty Years Later* (New York: Continuum, 1982), p. 13.

"Rank, whose imagination . . ."; Jones, *Life and Work,* vol. 3, p. 76.

"the wolves stood for his parents' white underwear"; *Coll. Papers,* vol. III, p. 515.

PSYCHOCULINARY DEVELOPMENT AND THE EATING CRISIS OF PUBERTY

After the peculiarities of early childhood appetites are surmounted, eating pleasures stabilize into a prolonged latency period of habitual tastes, only to break out again with a vengeance after the bar mitzvah. Possibly, the bar mitzvah party itself acts as an initiation ceremony into adolescent orgiastic eating. The great platters of chopped liver, of herring in cream, of whitefish and Nova Scotia salmon, the many breads . . . the family romance of mother and father, uncles and aunts, cousins of different appetites, all pressing their bodies closer and closer around the buffet, present a vivid introduction into mature adult eating, corresponding to the initiate's newly discovered and hugely increased physical hunger.

Before we can pursue our investigation into the critical changes that assault the human appetites at puberty, everafter affecting the person's entire psychoculinary development, we must once again, reader, go back to early childhood. You will recall that the formative years at table are subject to various traumas (q.v., "Totem and Tapioca," "The Primal Meal," "Oedipal Pie," "Deep-Dish Apple Trauma," etc.).♦ The main characteristics of these early years is the partiality of the eating drive—what I have previously termed "partial drives." The small child is partial only to certain foods and fiercely rejects others. He or she is a fussy eater: only orange juice and not grapefruit; only peanut butter and not peanuts; only eggs cooked harder than 5 minutes and not cracked; or an absurd dislike for good rye bread.

The second characteristic of childhood appetite is the polymorphous perversity of the eating drive. Peculiar, even perverse combinations are indulged in and always in the same obsessive way: mashed potatoes with grape jelly, catsup and matzo, or advanced cravings for Greek olives and Mexican hot sauce, all too sophisticated for a little palate.

These strong partialities and perversions nonetheless form the base of the gourmet's recipes. It is the fussy child that becomes the exacting taster. Psychoanalysis has established, incontrovertibly, that all later delicacies—sauces,

♦ No recipe for "Deep-Dish Apple Trauma" has been found.— *The Editors.*

marinades, forcemeats—owe their origins to the peculiar perversions of the child. What begins as a strange mixture in the highchair matures into the delicate pâtés of haute cuisine, but only if the child's exaggerations are not cut off at puberty, thereby diverting psychoculinary development into the neurotic paths of late adolescent eating disorders.

To guard against such later neuroses, it is advisable to remember my own case studies (cf., "The Wolfman's Easy Walnut Chicken," "The Ratman's Cheesecake," "Little Hansburgers," etc.). For, in puberty, we witness enactments of these classical models. Some at puberty show Wolfman appetites: whole small chickens, quarts of ice cream, milk chugged down by the half-gallon. Others repeat the behavior of a Ratman: sneaking into the larder on a surreptitious mission to seek and destroy whatever is lying around. The craving for Hansburgers and eating like a horse is too well known to be described.

The therapy of choice here is to lead the young person at puberty to the kitchen, not merely to eat or lay waste the refrigerator, but to cook; that is, to find ways to self-satisfy the exaggerated appetites by his own hand without guilt over their enormity.

Although I have here expounded upon the puberty crisis in the male, readers will surely recall the early female case studies (Dora, Anna O.) that provide hysterical examples of arrested psychoculinary development. Young women at puberty, in order to distinguish their gender from gross brothers greedily gulping, lapse into a picky disdain for food (like my case of Beth, "The Bird Girl") or they pig out away from home (like another recent case, Tracy, "The Pig Girl").

When psychoculinary development successfully passes through the puberty crisis, there occurs a gradual refinement of taste and the sublimating of perversions and partialities into interesting dinners in the discreet privacy of one's home. But should the eating crisis of puberty remain fixated, psychoculinary development takes a path that leads straight to those late adolescent disorders known as anorexia, obesity, and bulemia. Here begins that dementia praecox and disintegration of culture that is so widespread today: an addiction to Jung Food, to the illusions of Wonderbread, and to submergence in the black tide of occultism.

THE UNCANNY

It is only rarely that a psychoanalyst feels impelled to investigate canned goods. He works on other planes of gustatory pleasure and has little to do with those lifeless containers of tasteless morbidity. But this is a mistake: morbidity is where our calling lies.

Yet the "uncanny," as I wrote wistfully in 1919 just after the War when fresh foods were still unavailable, is for many a rather remote region and one that, as a subject for study, has been much neglected. The uncanny, for most of the world's people, still remains as I described it then, as belonging "to all that is terrible—to all that arouses dread and creeping horror."

For me it is just the opposite: nothing makes me shudder or disgusts me more than canned peas, canned soups, or canned fruit juices. Nor do I exclude frozen or embalmed foods: on a recent trip to France I was startled by the number of restaurants serving frozen *pommes frites* and by the number of Frenchmen, their palates equally frost-bitten, eating them.

What has happened? Why this constant fear of the uncanny? What can we as psychoanalysts do to get people to eat fresh fruits and vegetables, unbottled mayonnaise, fresh instead of tinned shrimp or salmon? I fear there is little we can do. For myself, it is even a matter of bitter recognition to realize how oversubtle my own writings in this regard have been, how I gave the public, and even my own disciples, too much credit for understanding the depths of the human psyche once I had explained them.

For instance, in my original piece on the uncanny, I offered what I thought was an enlightening view of the irony involved in *unheimlich* (uncanny) feelings: "It often happens that male patients declare that they feel there is something uncanny about the female genital organs. This *unheimlich* place, however, is the entrance to the former *heim* [home] of all human beings, to the place where everyone dwelt once-upon-a-time and in the beginning. There is a humorous saying: 'Love is home-sickness.'"

There it is, clear and even humorous. But do you think anyone understood what I was trying to say there about canned goods? Did I have to spell it out even more? Should I have issued engraved invitations to the human race announcing the happiness that comes from eating the truly uncanny?

I have been spat on, denounced, and maligned, but have I been read? Do even the so-called Freudians read my works anymore? All I was ever trying to do was offer miserable mankind a little pleasure, a little joy, in that otherwise wretched, meaningless, and self-punishing experience it calls life.

I am tempted to cry, Go on, humanity! Eat your canned spaghetti sauce, your powdered eggs and dried potato flakes, your bottled "French" salad dressings and microwaved frozen beef chips! But I cannot. I think only of your suffering every night as once again I prepare to wash the lettuce, peel the potatoes, and, for myself at least, start all things afresh.

NOTES

"to all that is terrible"; *Coll. Papers,* vol. IV, p. 368.
"It often happens"; *Coll. Papers,* vol. IV, p. 398.

H. W. FRINKFURTERS

These are not your normal American hotdogs but show the influence of true Wieners. H. W. Frink himself was not a Wiener; he came over from New York with that promising batch of younger professionals to learn from me after the Great War. Frink learned fast and I thought him the ablest American I had yet run across—I still do, even though he had that psychotic episode during the analysis, and a few years later lost sanity altogether, his life ending in a mental hospital in a place called North Carolina.

The menu at this institution seemed unduly limited: they served wieners every night. According to Frink it was because of some insane association the staff made between Vienna and psychoanalysis, as if Viennese food, or what they thought was Viennese food, namely, wieners, would help the patients. Frink tried to explain the nonsense of this, but did not get very far, inasmuch as he was himself a patient. Frink, further, sent me the following recipe which represents the institution's nightly dish, in the expectation that I would write to them and put an end to their folly. By the time I replied, unfortunately, he was dead. I do not, therefore, recommend H. W. Frinkfurters, though they are no doubt useful in mental hospitals that are overcrowded.

Mix thoroughly (!) 1 cup catsup, 1 cup water, and 1 tbs. vinegar. Add 1 tbs. sugar, 1 tbs. mustard, 1 tsp. curry powder, and 3 tbs. chopped onions. Simmer for 1/2 hour. Add a package of wieners and continue cooking for 15 minutes, or until all of the nitrites in the "meat" are active. Serve in the "sauce."

NOTE
"Frink learned fast . . .": Jones *Life and Work,* vol. 3, pp. 111–112.

BEEF THANATOS

Sooner or later everyone discovers it: the kitchen is a killer, a center for death or "Thanatos," as the Greeks called it. Thanatos represents the self-destructive instincts, as opposed to the life-instincts of Eros. Thanatos is behind our masochistic and sadistic behaviors, and nowhere more so than in the kitchen, whose two primary instruments are the knife and fire. Furthermore, it is the self-destructive instinct of Thanatos that governs oversalting and over-cooking, dropping the skillet on our toes, scalding our arms, and slicing our thumbs. And without Thanatos, who could approach the chopping block, cleaver in hand, or gut a hare, truss a bird, decapitate a fish, or even pick the eyes from an old potato?

Because of Thanatos I pay no attention to patients' complaints about sweating over a hot stove or the deadly ordeals of marketing. The joy of cooking is often hidden as a kitchen masochism. I say to such patients, If you cannot take the heat, stay out of the kitchen. A good patient, like a good cook, will not, or cannot; he or she always goes back for more.

> Beef Thanatos is, in spite of its name, more of an hors d'oeuvre than a finish. It is made with phyllo, a paper-thin dough used in Egyptian and Middle Eastern cooking. Cut the dough into several little squares and place a tsp. of beef filling in the center of each. Wrap other strips of phyllo around these, as if you were wrapping a mummy. Place on greased baking sheet and bake at 350° for about ½ hour or until brown. Serve warm, or freeze them (under proper cryogenic conditions, these hors d'oeuvres will keep for centuries). They are delicious as last-minute snacks for hungry patients, especially those with death fears.
> For the body of this dish, grind up (in food

processor) 3 or 4 cups leftover cooked beefsteak.

Saute ½ cup diced sweet peppers, and ½ cup chopped onion. Mix the vegetables in a bowl with the beef, and with ½ cup chopped parsley, ¼ cup feta cheese, 2 egg yolks, and a few sprigs of chopped mint.

PARANOID PIE

It is a striking feature in the behavior of paranoids that they attach the greatest significance to trivial details in other people's cooking. Details which are usually overlooked by others they interpret as the basis of some far-reaching culinary conclusions. For example, if you mix a little sour cream with the apples filling a pie, paranoids will ask, "Are you Jewish?" When you say no, they will say, "Did you think I was Jewish?" If you add to the apples in the pie a layer of finely chopped almonds (along with an egg, a little cream, brown sugar, and rum), they will remind you that cyanide smells like almonds too. If you simply fill a baked pie crust with cold applesauce (no matter how you spice it) and serve it cold, paranoids will ask, "Would you bake my piece to kill the bacteria?"

All that the paranoid observes is full of meaning. All is explainable, which is of course not true of good cooking, which relies so much on imagination. Paranoids, as everyone knows by now (but how long it took me to convince people!) project into the cookery of others whatever is cooking in their own unconscious. But one must be cautious—often the paranoid's behavior is justified: he perceives something that escapes the normal cook. "Is something burning?" he will ask, and you will say, "Oh, my god, the pie!" He sees clearer than cooks of normal intellectual capacity, but his knowledge is worthless when he starts imputing to others his own state of affairs.

Thus I have, over the years, devised the perfect dessert for such people, one that gives them no quarter in your kitchen: Paranoid Pie.

In a food processor, mix 2 cups flour, $1^1/_2$ tbs. granulated sugar and $1^1/_2$ tbs. brown sugar, 1 tsp. baking powder, and a suspicion of salt. Slowly add $^1/_2$ cup cream, $1^1/_2$ sticks butter, broken into bits, and 1 egg. When the dough forms a ball, take it out and knead by hand for a minute. Roll out the dough and cut into 2 pieces, for top and bottom. Fit the first piece in the bottom of a buttered pie pan. Fill the pie with nothing but fantasies, then fit the top piece over it. Trim edges, and bake in 375° oven for 10 minutes. Serve cool.

ON APHRODISIACS, OR BEYOND THE PLEASURE PRINCIPLE

An age-old human fantasy insists that certain victuals nourish the sexual drive—red meats, raw eggs, oysters, various chilis, absinthe, and now even parsley has joined the ranks of chosen foods whose direct effect is to furnish the sexual organs with more vitality and the sexual desire with more urgency. The correction that psychoanalysis has brought to this ancient superstition results from the discovery that the id, home of vital desires and source of pleasure, is always confronted with an equally powerful antagonist, the superego. A drive always meets an inhibition. Therefore, if with a tasty aphrodisiac we increase the volume of the drive, instead of achieving the desired goal of penile erection or vaginal lubricity or a more extended and intensified sexual performance, we succeed only in meeting a more stubborn denial, a more repressive inhibition from the superego.

Bowing before the superego's eternal condemnation of pleasure, psychoanalysis today reverses the aim of the aphrodisiac. Our concoctions aim instead at the superego itself, the carrier of the death instinct. We feed the death instinct—all the while knowing that the pleasurable cravings of the repressed id will return with revenge, claiming omnipotent satisfaction. To encourage the id, feed the superego.

The effective aphrodisiacs, then, are rye crisps, Finn crisps, pumpkin seeds, plain yogurts, dried dulse, sour rosehips and windfall apples. You cannot go wrong if you use whatever is shriveled, astringent, and gray. These aphrodisiacs are available in specialty shops (often near porn shops) called health food stores, which are nothing but disguised temples to the death instinct. In your search for aphrodisiacal pleasures, remember the formula: health food equals death food equals the raunchy revenge of the id.

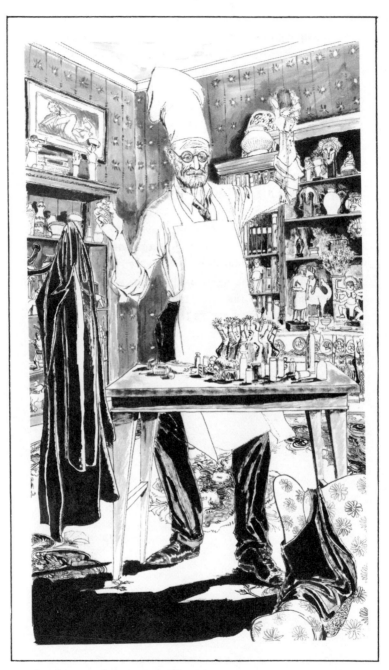

Megalomania Crown Roast of Lamb

X.

CARRY OUT, OR FOOD TO GO: MY FINAL RECIPES FOR HUMANITY♦

Including Wonderbread (or, The Future of an Illusion) and Freud Clams

"I sport a gardenia every day and act the rich man who lives only for his whims. Life will be serious soon enough. In any case it was wonderful while it lasted."
—Letter to Martha, 25 September 1912, in *The Letters of Sigmund Freud, 1873–1939*, ed. E. L. Freud

♦ Freud seems to have made no decision what to call this section of the manuscript, with all of the above, in various combinations, written and crossed out several times. The above is our own reconstruction. —*The Editors*

CIVILIZATION AND ITS INDIGESTION

I beg the reader's permission, at this point, to interject a theoretical consideration that arises from confusion brought on by the mistranslation of my work, *Das Unbehagen in der Kultur* (*Civilization and Its Discontents*), which should read *Discomfort in Culture*. As I maintained in chapter 4 of that work, cultural progress has been achieved at the cost of the sense of smell. The advance from smell to vision, the sacrifice of the olfactory in favor of the optic, is the fundamental source of cultural discomfort. The powerful frustration represented by the consumption of odorless and consequently tasteless meals, meals prepared for the eyes only, together with the repression of olfactory pleasures, results in that universal discomfort of our culture, indigestion. Indigestion, I now see, is more universal than the Oedipus complex. Earlier, I did not recognize how much everyone wishes for tasty meals; more, it seems, than those who find their mothers that appealing.

While we are pursuing this matter of translating my German into English, there is another title which the psychosquabbles (now, there is a dish I must prepare sometime) among Brill, Jones, and Strachey distorted. I refer to *Triebe und Triebschicksale,* which they translated "Instincts and Their Vicissitudes." It should simply have been translated "Drives and Their Destinies." *Triebe* means "drive" and *Schicksal* suggests *Schickse,* the pleasant Yiddish term for a non-Jewish young woman. The latent intention in my title would have thus become manifestly clear: our drives and destinies are determined by the fateful *Schickse.*

(Jung presumptuously rebaptized my discovery for the love object of men with his pompous Latinate term "Anima." This unabashed borrowing, or plagiarism, is revealed in his statement that the anima is a man's fate. *Wurst!* Jung's so-called anima is nothing but a *Schickse* in disguise.)

NEUROTIC STEW, OR OMNIPOTENCE TOPF: WHAT TO DO

The art of making a neurotic stew instead of falling or getting into one—that is the aim of psychoanalysis. The major components of the stew are of course whatever lies about—carrots, cabbage, potatoes; the children, your sister-in-law, your pets. But the art of a neurotic stew lies in decisive combinations. Here the Fates intervene with obsessive scruples. The neurotic personality becomes unable to separate this from that, what to put in first and what later, whether sliced or halved, cumin or caraway. As the mess steams up, vision clouds, and the slow boil (so essential to a good stew) becomes furiously turbulent, eventually blowing the lid. The patient loses sight of what's in the pot, why he or she is doing this in the first place, and throws the stew out with the dishwater. The patient has fallen into a neurotic stew.

Just here lies the difference between the neurotic stew and the Omnipotence *Topf.* Into the *Topf* anything goes, head first, headlong. Turkey wings? Sure. Frozen *pois mange tout,* heavy beef, some sherry—why not? To the Omnipotence *Topf* everything belongs, so there are no decisions, whereas the neurotic stew is an agony of choices swiftly accompanied by undoings, with attempts to salvage what is already parboiled. The neurotic stew therefore defeats analysis. It is an incurable condition because irreversible: we cannot restore the *status quo ante* once the potatoes have softened and the cabbage fallen apart.

Thus prevention is the psychoanalytic treatment: we must prevent the original fall into the stew in the first place and not fruitlessly try to take it apart once it has begun to steam up. The art is medical: a prescription is called for and must be followed exactly. One must have a list of ingredients, their proper sizes, measurable quantities, schedule of timings. The patient must be given no occasion for choices along the way. The art of the stew builds a strong ego. It is a work of culture.

FREUD'S FAMOUS FAIRY-TALE COOKIES

Cookies! I should have made more cookies! Gingerbread cookies were especially helpful with patients who did not understand what was going on in the fairy tales of childhood. For example, the young American patient of whom I reported in my study, *Inhibitions, Symptoms and Anxiety:* "His sexual excitement had been kindled by a fantastic nursery tale which was read to him of an Arab sheik who pursued a Gingerbread Man in order to devour him. With this edible being he identified himself . . . and this fantasy became the first substratum of his autoerotic activity." First substratum indeed! Now I can say openly, a couple of properly shaped gingerbread cookies and the boy was fine.

Human nature always seeks to allay anxiety, behind which lies the childhood fear of being eaten (see "Little Hansburgers"). You would think a good cookie is all it would take to get over this fear. But the formula, Child = Edible Cookie, creates such anxiety that it converts into the cookie compulsion. By eating the cookie, we are saved from being devoured. (See "Wonderbread, or the Future of an Illusion"). Cookie anxiety and cookie compulsion thus follow Darwin's great law of evolution: eat or be eaten.

A cookie a day keeps anxiety away—and even the finest available would be less costly to the household budget than the incredible cost today of analysis five times a week. Patients, in fact, used to tell me that I should have gone into the cookie business, my own famous fairy-tale cookies were that good (probably because children were not used to this much brandy in their cookies).

Cut the gingerbread cookies into the shape of men and women, boys and girls, and even animals. One can be a gingerbread man. Another can be in the shape of Hansel, whom the witch, in the famous fairy tale, was fattening up to eat, and who used to stick his, well, "finger" out every day for her to see if it was "fat enough" yet. And you can make one of Little Red Riding Hood, whom the wolf was going to, well, "eat" too. If you do make a wolf, make him big.

> Mix 2 sticks of softened butter, $1/2$ cup brown sugar, 2 eggs, $1/4$ cup molasses, $1/2$ glass of German Branntwein (or any brandy you prefer), 1 tbs. ginger, $1/2$ tbs. nutmeg, 1 tsp. baking soda, 1 tsp. cinnamon, and about 4 cups flour (batter should not be sticky). When the dough is rolled, cut into thin shapes with your cookie molds, and place on buttered baking sheet. Bake in 350° oven for about 10 minutes, until just beginning to brown (the centers will be soft because of the brandy).

NOTE
"His sexual excitement . . ."; *The Problem of Anxiety*, trans. Henry Alden Bunker (New York: Norton, 1963), p. 34.

HILDA DOOLITTLE'S MOTHER'S PANCAKES

The American poet who called herself H.D. came to me in the 1930s to be cured of fears she had about being abandoned. It was a simple case of freeing her from an early mother fixation. She never did understand this: I had to get her to refuse to accept even my own interpretations in order to free her from her mother. Hilda and her goddesses! (She was born in Bethlehem, Pennsylvania, and never got over the coincidence.) How she resisted! Even in her later "Tribute" to me, she insisted that there was "an argument implicit in our very bones" and that I was not always right. Well, I was right about one thing: she made good pancakes.

> Take 1 cup of boiled, mashed squash (the
> Pennsylvania Dutch influence, I believe), add 1 cup of
> boiling milk along with 1 tbs. butter, 1 tbs. sugar, and
> the barest initial of salt. Cool it! Pretend you are
> abandoning the batter altogether. Then come back
> and add 1 well-beaten egg, 1 tsp. baking powder, and
> 1 cup of flour. Spoon the batter onto a hot greased
> griddle, putting one spoonful in the middle and
> several sibling spoonfuls around the side. When they
> bubble, turn them. They are done in a second, as
> quick as you can say—H.D.!

WHAT DO THEY WANT? WHAT DO THEY WANT?

> *". . . the logic of soup, with dumplings for arguments."*

To this day, as I have often said, I "cannot solve the riddle of femininity" despite devoting many chapters of my writings and many hours of my practice to the psychology of woman. In my early years, and while still under the influence of Parisian teachers, I believed the right diet for the female of our species consisted in such dishes as popovers, *concombres farcis,* pork sausage, *coq au vin,* walnuts and figs, or even thick white Cavaillon asparagus (see also "Banana O.").

As my studies penetrated more deeply into female sexuality, I recognized that something still seemed to be wanted, something more elusive, like sweetbreads and truffles, or a *consommé aux cheveux d'ange.* Further revision of psychoanalytic theory brought us to realize the significance of the mother in forming the little girl's character, so that menu choice (or object choice as we used to call it) of the mature woman may very well turn to homemade biscuits, baked apples with warm milk, thick velouté soups, and lovingly prepared vegetables of all kinds, especially multifoliate florals such as cabbage and cauliflower.

What did become certain in the course of time was a definition of what women did not want: the castrated foods of women's luncheons: raspberry tinted butter, sweet poppyseed dressings, little timbales of rice without spice, meat without bones, bread without crust, queen-sized portions in cosmetic colors on dainty doilies of *fraises rêve de bébé.* Why must women sit at too-small tables on too-small chairs with too-small napkins eating oversized desserts? Female foods have yet to be investigated in terms of the Goldilocks syndrome.

Some years back I wrote, "I too didn't much like Frau Dr. Fr. Perhaps I'm doing her an injustice when I classify her as meat dish: 'goose'; vegetable dish: *zwidderwurzen.*" Now I am convinced that I was not doing her an injustice at all. I was paying her a compliment.

But what do they want? What do they want? Because the answer still escapes us, we should not pretend to know what we do not know, and so I offer no recipe for what women want. I can only repeat, "If you want to know more about femininity, you must interrogate your own experience, or turn to the poets or else wait until science can give you more profound and more coherent information."

NOTES

"the logic of soup"; "Observations on transference-love," *Standard Edition,* 12 (London: Hogarth Press, 1958), p. 159. See also K. R. Eissler, *Talent and Genius* (New York: Quadrangle, 1971), p. 256.
"cannot solve the riddle of femininity"; "The Psychology of Women," *New Introductory Lectures on Psycho-Analysis,* 33, trans. W. J. H. Sprott (London: Hogarth, 1933), p. 149.
"if you want to know"; ibid., p. 174.
"I too didn't much like Frau Dr. Fr."; Max Schur, op. cit., p. 47.

WILHELM REICH AND ORGONIC CEREALS

I never took stock in health food—what could be healthier than our regular *Mittagessen* with good Viennese fare? But quack ideas, reducing the psyche to the body, plagued me from every side. I was surrounded by nothing but nuts and quackers. First Fliess and the nose rhythms, then Adler and his organ inferiority, then Groddeck, and finally Reich.

Poor Reich. Many of my followers met unusual fates. I think of Abraham and the fishbone, of Tausk and Silberer dead at their own hands, of Hermine Hug-Hellmuth murdered by her nephew, a patient. But to end up as Reich did, in a federal penitentiary in Pennsylvania, for mail fraud, does this not show the power of the death instinct over the life of one who so single-mindedly insisted upon Eros?

Reich first came to me in 1919 or 1920, a medical student only twenty-three years old. We took to each other at once, and I soon sent him a patient. My timorous Viennese followers could not abide his radical politics and were not pleased at having yet another paranoid character in their midst. Besides, he was fascinated with sex, even more than they were. He even called his autobiography *Function of the Orgasm*—yet are we not each the end product of just this function?

I used to think—we all used to think—that it was from studying the orgasm that he developed his crackpot orgone theory. Now I read in a biography of him (it is all I can do anymore to keep up with the biographies of my disciples) that his orgones came from a cook pot.

While searching around one day for the cosmic force, or orgone energy, "He bought meat, vegetables, eggs and milk, put them all in a saucepan, and boiled up the mixture for half an hour. Then he took a drop of this soup and placed it under the microscope. What he saw on the slide took his breath away—myriad globules moving in every direction. He immediately came to the conclusion that these globules were full of biological energy and that he had found what he was looking for."

What he was looking for, apparently, was the *bion* or fundamental unit of the orgone. He called his treatment vegetotherapy and put himself and his patients into orgone boxes to capture the rays of the universe. What a *meshugana!*

But try orgonic cereals for thirty days and see if they do not make you feel better. If only Reich had stayed with these, and worked on a good orgonic cereal box, perhaps with an athlete pictured on it, he could have been a rich man.

NOTE

"He bought meat . . ."; Michael Cattier, *The Life and Work of Wilhelm Reich,* trans. Ghislaine Boulanger (New York: Avon, 1971), p. 197.

MEGALOMANIA CROWN ROAST OF LAMB

This recipe I give entirely as I received it from the pen of Wilhelm Reich:

> Let go! Buy a whole crown roast from your butcher! Tip your butcher! Put on a chef's hat! Turn your oven up to 500°! Season the crown with salt and pepper and rosemary sprigs and everything else you have in your herb collection! Stuff the crown with a mixture of 2 tsp. sage, 2 tbs. chopped onion, parsley, chervil, thyme, coriander, and whatever else you want. It is your crown roast, baby! Then come to your senses. Do you really want your roast to go up in flames?
>
> Place on roaster rack and bake, uncovered, at 300° for 15 to 20 minutes per pound or even less depending on desired rareness. But have it very rare! And instead of the usual paper frills over rib ends, try ten-dollar bills! You can still fulfill your delusions of grandeur without burning down the house!

THE TRANSFERENCE COUNTER

I wish we had known about the transference counter in the early days. It would have saved us all a lot of trouble. Breuer would not have been so disturbed by Anna O. that a sudden escape to Venice seemed called for; Jung would have better understood his affair with Sabina Spielrein; and some would say that even I, vis-à-vis my association with Tausk, might have been more circumspect (in this latter case, I do not agree—I never felt anything for Tausk, except on our salad days).

We used to just cook along and put what was too hot to handle back into the patient's hands (without even so much as a potholder), and call the patient's objections "the transference." That is, we transferred problems now appearing in the analysis back into the patient's own kitchen or into his family's kitchen of childhood.

This problem was especially hard to handle for nonmedical analysts. They did not have the skill which physicians enjoy of laying things onto the patient so as to protect themselves. I analyzed this problem in my essay, *The Question of Lay Analysis,* so that my nonmedical colleagues would not be regarded as inferior.

The problem was a serious one. But, as fortune favors the brave, so time has favored our science, always forcing it to new inventions. The transference proved too painful: the patient, too, had to have a place to put his hot potatoes. And so we devised the transference counter. Analysts nowadays are trained especially in its construction. It must not be flammable, it must be smoothly surfaced—no rough edges that catch projections—and it must be low enough so the stuff laid out on it can be seen into. If the transference counter is set up right, no one will get burned. Clearly a must for the smart kitchen!

MOSES AND MATZOBALLISM

I confess to a long-standing affection for the matzoball, perhaps for its ease in swallowing whole. The small round form, always fashioned by hand, passed over with the Israelites when they fled Egypt. There, the round sun-disc with hands provided the model for the original, or Ur, matzoball of Pharaoh Akhenaten. It thus recalls some of the earliest culinary culture of humankind. My controversial book, *Moses and Monotheism,* brought evidence to show that the matzoball is not a Jewish invention, but Egyptian, as was Moses himself. To those speculations, I would now add one more: Moses was slow of speech, as the Bible says, not because Hebrew was not his tongue, but because he had burned it schlurping matzoball soup.

For me the little ball, uniform, supportive, and immersed in its bowl of broth, answers to the deepest needs of mankind for a universal symbol in its struggle for meaning. The matzoball, compact and indissoluble, is the ego in the midst of the primal broth. No sublimations are permitted: it may not be too light so that it floats. No substitutions either: it may not be made of bread crumbs instead of matzo. Above all, there must only be the one.

MELANIE KLEIN'S GOOD AND BAD BREASTS OF CHICKEN

"The desire of the child for its first form of nourishment is altogether insatiable . . . it never gets over the pain of losing the mother's breast." I was always satisfied with that observation until Mrs. Klein came along and complicated it all. Not one breast but two! she said. Not one emotion but two! Not just the good breast of nourishing but the bad breast of weaning. Now there was the withholding mother, the mother who feeds her other children, provoking rivalry, envy, ambivalence. *Oy,* so many complications— that's what "neo"-Freudianism means, it means more complications! Imagine, people become "Kleinians" so they can tell a good breast from a bad.

I say, when it comes to chicken, *keine Sorge* (no problem)! In this recipe, it is easy to watch out for ambivalence; one will have no trouble distinguishing which breast is which. Just be sure you make enough. Each guest must be served a boneless double breast of chicken. One breast is covered with a Mexican *mole* sauce, the other with a

Nordic cream (Swedish sour cream). Guests may turn their plates at will to eat first the breast they prefer.

> For the *mole* sauce, which should be of a thick consistency, blend several ground black chilies (seeded) with 1 oz. of bittersweet chocolate, and 3 cups of hot chicken broth.
> For the Nordic cream, combine 1 cup sour cream, 1 tbs. finely grated fresh horseradish, 1 tbs. fresh dill, and a dash of salt. Chill before serving on the chicken.

NOTE
"The child's avidity . . ."; "Femininity," *New Introductory Lectures on Psycho-Analysis,* trans. W. J. H. Sprott, p. 156.

WONDERBREAD, OR THE FUTURE OF AN ILLUSION

My theory of bread lay all but dormant on a shelf for half a century. It rose slowly into consciousness after its first infusion with Breuer's yeast in 1881, derived from that famous encounter with the passion of his patient, Anna O. When she flung her arms around his neck, why did he run away? What impairment of passion had so affected his instinctual body that this normal and altogether genuine show of affection struck him with a fear unto death? On that decisive morning so many years ago what had he had for breakfast? Toast?

Prolonged inquiry (carried out with the greatest caution so as not to evoke hysteria in the Breuer family) established that he had taken, as usual, a continental breakfast consisting of a Gipfel or two and other little rolls of refined flour. His course of action in the consulting room had been prepared unconsciously at the break of day: Breuer was fatefully reenacting the instinctual renunciation going on daily in the bakeries and homes of an entire civilization: its religious addiction to white bread.

Bread was also Anna's incurable symptom. Breuer reported: "She allowed me to feed her, so that she very soon began to take more food. But she never consented to eat bread. After her meal she invariably rinsed out her mouth." Clearly, Anna's symptom was an attempt at cure, a *cri du coeur:* she wanted her instincts back. Wanting a healthy body instead of all her crazy symptoms, her unconscious mind knew that the kind of bread Breuer ate was a source of illness. She would not touch it.

In our German language the association between bread and body is only too plain. The same word-sound means body (*Leib*) and loaf (*Laib*). So, an overrefined loaf equals an instinctless body. Both doctor and patient were afflicted by a disease in the culture—its daily breads. If a whole culture suffers, can an individual be spared? No psychoanalytic wonder-cure can cure this plague of wonderbread.

Only after I had passed through several death crises myself and reached the other side of my seventies did I dare link civilization's bread neurosis to religion outright. None other than Jesus says (John 6:51) "I am the living bread . . . the bread . . . is my flesh." In fact, Jesus and his *companions* (the word derives from *panis,* bread, and means that they ate bread with each other) do a lot of talking about bread. It makes the serious student of the Bible wonder if all the emphasis on Jesus the carpenter or his cronies the fishermen is not but a disguise for the fact that they were really in the bread business, producing loaves out of thin air for a multitude of customers.

Thus the refining process in the flour mills, which castrates the wheat of its germinating seed, is a secondary elaboration of our culture's theology whose God of salvation has no mature genitality. Simply put, bread will be soppy on earth so long as sappiness rules in heaven. Those dead white loaves turned out on endless belts (the technology of eternity), attended by acolytes and ministrants in white, can never age, never stale, only chemically decompose. The limp, doughy bodies, embalmed with gaseous bubbles (for yeast takes its own natural time) and injected with a cryptic litany of esoteric additives, their outer faces cosmeticized with caramel (for such bread does not darken in heat or form a crust), emerge risen and ethereal in minutes (it is instant resurrection), each body covered with its plastic Veil of Turin, a slippery, soggy, sentimental sublimation, all passion spent.

When Nietzsche said "God is dead," he had just been served a slice of wonderbread by his sister, and, his mouth crammed with an unswallowable gulp of the stuff, she misheard what he was trying to say. Never imagining that a diseased mind like her brother's could make an intelligent comment about what he was eating, she transcribed his remark on the demise of bread as yet another of his attacks on deity. Poor Nietzsche. He was never understood.

In the same way, some decided that my book on wonderbread (*The Future of an Illusion*) was a deliberate attack on the illusion of salvation in "white Christian civilization." That good Swiss Protestant, Pastor Pfister (see "Veal Oskar Pfister") wrote a refutation. But these critics, as always with my work, missed the point: I was not out to get salvation, I was only trying to save bread.

My investigation into bread, therefore, had to go all the way. This meant into its roots in religion, for wonderbread is merely the end product of a long cultural evolution, a religious evolution. The bread that was the god (primitive identification), and the breaking of the loaf that was the god's body (totemism) and then the sharing of that broken bread in a communal meal commemorated with different Christian masses (sacrifice of the father imago) became sublimated over time into the neurosis of civilization, resulting in that little tasteless wafer, a mere macaroon or meringue without savor or crumb; bleached, stamped, boxed, and slipped onto the id-less penitent's tongue in uniform sterile portions that next became uniform slices of "bread for the masses."

The illusion we now call "bread" has no future. Nor does the civilization that comes wrapped with it. As long as the prayer goes forth daily to Mister Muffin Man in the Sky to give us this day our daily bread, our flour mills will go on grinding and bleaching, our loaves knowing neither ferment nor crust, and our sandwiches dwelling forever in the house of gumminess and goo.

No, the bagel is not the answer. Nor is Vienna bread. No matter how they twist it into ever new-fangled Freudian shapes, these are just fancier versions of the same white civilized flour.

I offer no recipe for bread. Why should an old man? Have I not done enough already? But advice I do have: if you would live as long as I, if you want a future that is not an illusion, get yourself a nice loaf of Jewish rye. Enjoy!

NOTES

"she allowed me to feed her"; Josef Breuer, "Studies on Hysteria," "Case 1, Fraulein Anna O.," *Standard Edition,* vol. II, pp. 26–27.
"white Christian civilization"; *The Future of an Illusion,* trans. W. D. Robson-Scott and James Strachey (New York: Anchor Books, 1964), p. 28.

FREUD CLAMS

The cherrystone, so to speak, of all psychoanalytic practice is a remarkable paradox: the patient must freely associate, saying everything that comes into his mind as the tide there goes out, digging, raking, dredging up every deep burrower he can find, whether Little Neck or long, soft-shell or hard, while the analyst must withhold his reaction, sometimes passing the hour in complete silence, waiting, as it were, to serve up his little *Venus mercenaria* only when her half-shell is good and ready.

Every Freudian analysis is thus an open and shut case: the patient open, the analyst shut. The necessity to snaffle that Pismo, as they say here at the *Hungaria,* I have frequently characterized in my writings as the technique of frustration, abstention, or withholding. Every now and then, however, a patient will attempt to pry us open by direct questioning or other, more seductive maneuvers designed to catch us offguard like some lumbering geoduck with its siphon out. My caution in such cases remains ever as it was: "to conduct ourselves upon the model of the man-servant who has a single answer to every question or objection: 'All will come clean in the course of future developments.' " In short, clam up!

That humble bivalve should thus have a place of honor in every psychoanalyst's office, alongside my bust, my portrait, or my autograph. Barring that, let the analyst regularly, at intervals, dine on my fried clams—not, I must insist at once, those monstrous denizens of the deep fryer that come reburied in corn meal and flour.

> Freud Clams are drained, then quickly tossed by the pintful into a skillet, allowed a brief time of free association with a melted stick of butter, then just as quickly removed from the pan and seasoned the Viennese way, with paprika and parsley. American analysts may add a cautious spoonful of G. Stanley Hall's Worcester Sauce.

NOTE

"to conduct ourselves"; "Constructions in Analysis," *Coll. Papers,* vol. V, p. 367.

EATING OUT

It is a commonplace in psychoanalysis that we help the patient to "work through" and not "act out" his conflicts. In recent years, however, I have come to insist on an even more exact notion of this concept: we must help the patient, I now see, to work through and not to eat out.

In this connection, I call attention once again to the symbol of the restaurant in dreams, a symbol one must not overlook. If the café has a significant name, a special decor, or refers to a place famous for erotic assignations, then it is an easy symbol to decipher. Always concealed, however, in the manifest dining place is a childhood reminiscence of a singularly exciting meal (one's first chocolate mousse, for example), a meal laden with trauma or a traumatic episode (snapping bits of turtle in the soup).

Thus eating out becomes, in the adult life of neurotics, a substitution: an attempt to recapitulate the heightened emotions of childhood. The neurotic eats out rather than cooks at home. He does not believe he can be nourished by his own resources. Gratification must come from without, and so eating out rightly belongs among the more subtle defense mechanisms that keep the neurotic from his own kitchen.

What psychoanalysis calls "working through" must be seen as an effort to work through a new recipe. Furthermore, the perplexing riddle that I addressed in my paper, "Analysis Terminable or Interminable," solves itself: those patients who no longer eat out no longer need analysis. Cooking is the cure, and the occasional visit to the restaurant is merely to taste that rare dish one has not seen, and may never see, in cookbooks.

There is yet another aspect to this dilemma, however—one that is apparent from the title alone of a forthcoming paper of mine, "Cookbooks: Terminable or Interminable?"

There I elaborate further on this subject, but the lay reader by now will probably have made up his own mind on the matter, and in this case, though it is against all my instincts as an analyst to admit it, he will probably be correct.

INDEX

Boldface entries indicate recipes.